The Making of Global Health
Governance

The Making of Global Health Governance

China and the Global Fund to Fight AIDS,
Tuberculosis, and Malaria

Nicole A. Szlezák

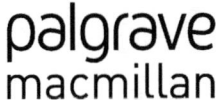

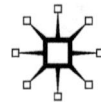

First published in 2012 by
PALGRAVE MACMILLAN®
in the United States—a division of St. Martin's Press LLC,
175 Fifth Avenue, New York, NY 10010.

Where this book is distributed in the UK, Europe and the rest of the World,
this is by Palgrave Macmillan, a division of Macmillan Publishers Limited,
registered in England, company number 785998, of Houndmills,
Basingstoke, Hampshire RG21 6XS.

Palgrave Macmillan is the global academic imprint of the above
companies and has companies and representatives throughout the world.

Palgrave® and Macmillan® are registered trademarks in the United
States, the United Kingdom, Europe and other countries.

ISBN: 978–1–137–02082–6

Library of Congress Cataloging-in-Publication Data

Szlezák, Nicole A., 1972–
    The making of global health governance : China and the global fund to
    fight AIDS, tuberculosis, and malaria / Nicole A. Szlezák.
        p.   cm.
    ISBN 978–1–137–02082–6 (hardback)
    1. World health.   2. Public health—International cooperation.
    3. Medical policy.   4. AIDS (Disease)—Social aspects.
    5. Tuberculosis—Social aspects.   6. Malaria—Social aspects.   I. Title.
    RA441.S96 2012
    362.1—dc23   2012011136

A catalogue record of the book is available from the British Library.

Design by Integra Software Services

First edition: September 2012

Contents

List of Tables

Author's Note

My motivation for writing this book goes back a long way. A physician by training, I worked in tropical medicine research for a brief period of my life, conducting biomedical research on malaria at the Albert Schweitzer Hospital in Lambaréné, Gabon. The work provided me, for a short time, with the humbling opportunity to be part of an entirely different world. I was struck by the contrast between the daily reality of my malaria patients, mostly primary school children, who lacked the most basic things including clean water and basic pediatric services, and the reality of a European biomedical researcher, contributing to a global body of knowledge about malaria, who could step into that world, and out again, at her own discretion.

A number of questions stirred my interest, which form the underlying structure of this book. Whose problems get the world's attention, and why? How do policy issues come to be regarded as global? How do new approaches to solving them gain currency and become accepted, financed, and implemented? And do new ways of framing things really lead to different ways of engagement? My search for intellectual tools to help me grapple with these questions led me to pursue a PhD at Harvard University's John F. Kennedy School of Government. Drawing on the multiple disciplinary perspectives inhabiting the School, I found myself drawn to study the emergence of *the global,* or *the transnational;* to observe its taking form as a set of rules and institutions; to follow its deployment into the real world; and to study its engagement with *the local.*

In this book I explore these themes through a focus on the Global Fund to Fight Aids, Tuberculosis and Malaria and its interaction with one of its largest grant recipients, China. In order to accomplish this task, I needed to follow a wide range of diverse threads, such as the emergence of HIV/AIDS as a global issue, changing paradigms driving international health cooperation, the evolution of ethical norms for global clinical trials, the emergence of trade and intellectual property regimes in the context of global pharmaceutical policy, the controversies around *AIDS denialism,* the emergence of the Global Fund as a new form of governance, the simultaneous emergence of several different HIV/AIDS epidemics in China, the changing image of HIV/AIDS in Chinese public perception and policy design, and, finally, the interaction between the Global Fund and China.

To make visible, trace, and connect these different themes, I relied on a wide array of materials—scientific literature, policy documents, newspaper articles, interviews, and first-hand testimonies of individuals in China and elsewhere. At the end of the book, the reader will find a long list of sources that were indispensable for the completion of this work. In addition to that, however, I would like to place on record my debt to three sources on which I relied especially heavily. Barton Gellman's excellent account of the political struggles surrounding the international community's approach to HIV/AIDS and the trade disputes surrounding the prices of antiretroviral medicines at the end of the 1990s, described in a series of articles in *The Washington Post* in 2000, was instrumental to me in understanding the changes in international norms—trade, intellectual property, and science—that preceded the creation of the Global Fund. I build on his work in large parts of Chapter 4. Edmund Settle's report *Aids in China: An Annotated Chronology 1985–2003* was tremendously helpful in gaining an overview of the major threads and milestones I needed to trace in order to understand how HIV/AIDS emerged and was conceptualized in China. One of these threads was that of the emergence of a so-called *plasma economy* in central China—a blood donation industry through which the HIV/AIDS virus was systematically spread to thousands of China's poorest citizens in Central China during the early 1990s. Direct testimony from these regions is hard to come by. Here, Zhang Ke's *Report on AIDS in Henan After a 5-Year Investigation* allowed me to understand the extent to which this entirely preventable epidemic was a direct consequence of local economic policy, and how government repression contributed to its severity and spread. I draw on his testimony on multiple occasions in chapters 5 and 6.

In discussing the formative interactions between the Global Fund and China, this book focuses on the period between 2002 and 2006. It is during this period that China submitted six HIV/AIDS grant applications to the Fund. Tracing these submissions allows us to witness an astonishing paradigm change from an approach that essentially proposed circumscribed, targeted prevention efforts in select subpopulations to a broad and inclusive national HIV/AIDS policy offering access to antiretroviral therapy to patients in need and proposing to actively engage grassroots civil society organizations. As I lay out in Chapter 7, the relationship between China and the Fund during that period shaped not only China's HIV/AIDS policy but also the Fund itself, and the broader concept of global health. Both the Fund and the idea of global health have, of course, continued to evolve since then, but the fundamentals have not changed.

Many people have supported me in writing this book. First and foremost, I thank my thesis advisors, Sheila Jasanoff, William Clark, and Anthony Saich, who led me through the process of researching and writing this work. It is with their intellectual guidance and continued support that I was able to assemble and connect the different threads that make up its substance. I also thank the Center for International Development and the Sustainability Science Program at Harvard for providing me with the resources and intellectual space that I needed to pursue this project. Finally, I thank many teachers and colleagues who helped me in multiple ways—by being thought partners in the design and implementation of this research, introducing me to interviewees, pointing me to valuable resources, and critiquing my writing—Lorrae van Kerkhoff, Suerie Moon, Joan Kaufmann, Arnold Howitt, Michael Hsu, and Kathrine Meyers.

Finally, I thank my family and my friends, without whom I could not have completed this work. Special thanks go to my friend Avi Kremer, whose courage and determination in the face of ALS continue to inspire me.

NICOLE A. SZLEZÁK

Abbreviations and Acronyms

3-TC	2',3'-dideoxy-3'-thiacytidine, an antiretroviral drug also called Lamivudine (brand name Epivir)
AIDS	Acquired Immune Deficiency Syndrome
ARV	Antiretroviral
AZT	Azidothymidine
BCG	Bacille Calmette Guerin
CBD	Commercial Blood Donors
CCM	Country Coordinating Mechanism
CDC	Centers for Disease Control
China CARES	China Comprehensive Aids RESponse
CNY	Chinese Yuan
CPT	Consumer Project on Technology
CSW	Commercial Sex Workers
D4T	Didehydro-deoxythymidine, an antiretroviral drug also called stavudine (brand name Zerit)
ddI	Didanosine
DFID	UK Department for International Development
DOTs	Directly Observed Tuberculosis Therapy, short course
FPD	Former Plasma Donors
GAVI	Global Alliance for Vaccines and Immunization
GDEP	Global DOTS Expansion Plan
GFATM	The Global Fund to Fight Aids, Tuberculosis and Malaria
GONGOs	Government-organized NGOs
GPA	WHO's Global Program on AIDS
GPSTB	Global Plan to Stop TB
GPT	Global Program on Tuberculosis at WHO
HIV	Human Immune Deficiency Virus

IUATLD	International Union Against Tuberculosis and Lung Disease
LFA	Local Fund Agent
MDR-TB	Multi-drug-resistant Tuberculosis
MSF	Medecins sans Frontieres
MSM	Men Who Have Sex with Men
MTCT	Mother-to-Child Transmission of HIV
PR	Principal Recipient
STDs	Sexually Transmitted Diseases
STIs	Sexually Transmitted Infections
TB	Tuberculosis
The Global Fund	The Global Fund to Fight Aids, Tuberculosis and Malaria
TRIPS	Trade-Related Aspects of Intellectual Property Rights
TRP	The Global Fund's Technical Review Panel
TWG	Transitional Working Group
UNAIDS	United Nations Programme on HIV/AIDS
UNDP	United Nations Development Program
UNFPA	United Nations Population Fund
UNICEF	United Nations Children's Fund
VCT	Voluntary Counseling and Testing
WTO	World Trade Organization

CHAPTER 1

Globalizing Public Policy: The Health Sector

March 2002 witnessed an important event in the history of international health: the Global Fund to Fight Aids, Tuberculosis and Malaria announced its first round of funding (Ramsay 2002). This was the first time that developing countries were able to access a billion-dollar Fund to support their efforts to address three long-standing health issues of utmost seriousness. In face of the threat posed by HIV/AIDS to people everywhere, the world, it seemed, had stopped and taken a breath. It had decided to depart from "business as usual" and to defy the socioeconomic divide between North and South, which commonly determines whether or not a person whose life is threatened by devastating illness will get access to life-saving treatment. The stakes were high, as were the hopes for the new organization.

The Global Fund was conceived of as a new kind of organization, one that will "not belong to one set of countries, or be tied to the United Nations, the World Bank or other institutions," but would be a "genuinely international entity" and also, at the same time, a "partnership between the public and private sector" (World Health Organization 2002a). Although the rich countries of the world dominate the health policy agenda, along with several other priorities, the Fund promises to allow developing countries to shape the response to some of their most pressing problems, with the support—yet without interference—of richer countries, and through a partnership among governments, the private sector, civil society, patients and their representatives, and the Fund itself.

The creation of the Global Fund illustrates larger trends of globalization at work in the world today. Increasing connectivity in trade, finance, and communications is leading to growing political, economic, and cultural integration. At the same time, certain problems are increasingly conceived of as "transnational" in the sense that they do not stay confined to the geographical or political spaces of individual nation-states—HIV/AIDS, climate change, and migration are prominent examples. Along with the view that some problems transcend national boundaries has come a perception that existing institutions, which are based on principles of national sovereignty and international cooperation, are inadequately equipped to solve those problems. Alternative models of governance are needed (Reinicke 1997; Nye and Donahue 2000; Brundtland 2002; Martens 2003.). The world is witnessing a gradual shift away from the traditional system of governance, which relied on governments, and intergovernmental organizations alone toward a system in which multiple actors, both state and nonstate, are playing an increasingly active role.

These trends are particularly visible in the health sector. Not only epidemics like HIV/AIDS and SARS (severe acute respiratory syndrome) but also noncommunicable health problems such as tobacco-related illnesses and cardiovascular diseases are increasingly viewed as global problems. Since the mid-1990s, more than a hundred new health organizations have emerged, independent of the multilateral institutions (Cohen 2006). Their missions vary, from the development of vaccines and drugs for diseases affecting developing countries to the provision of health care to patients in the poorest regions of the world (Widdus 2001, 2005). Some of these organizations are foundations, like the mighty Bill and Melinda Gates Foundation, which has billions at its disposal for research and development of new treatments for diseases that disproportionately affect the poor. Others are not-for-profit organizations, such as the Medicines for Malaria Venture or the Global Alliance for TB Drug Development, which strive to bring new malaria and tuberculosis drugs to the market. A majority of these new players, including most prominently the Global Fund to Fight Aids, Tuberculosis and Malaria, conceive of themselves in some way as "global partnerships" between the public and private sectors.

The idea that partnerships represent a superior way of cooperation marks a departure from traditional public health approaches. International health cooperation as first conceived in the mid-nineteenth century was built on the foundations of the Westphalian regime of 1648, which has governed relations among states for three centuries (Fidler 2003). Three principles are central to that regime. First, states are the primary actors in the international domain; second, rules are designed to address the interaction among states (such as rules of diplomacy, war, and trade); third, these rules should not interfere in the internal workings of states, that is, in the ways that national governments govern their territories and populations (Fidler 2003). International public health cooperation had its origins in 1849, after cholera epidemics had killed tens of thousands of Europeans (McCarthy 2002). In line with Westphalian principles, the goals and rules of international health protection were designed to control infectious diseases to advance trade and travel among (mainly European) sovereign states, and not to improve the health of all human beings (Fidler 2003).

Since the beginning of the twentieth century, international public health cooperation has gradually moved away from its Westphalian origins. This is true with respect to both primary policy goals and the interactions among different players in that domain. Thus, the proclaimed aim of international health policy is no longer limited to the prevention of epidemics, but to improve the health of all human beings on Earth, as evidenced in the World Health Organization's (WHO) 1978 Declaration of Alma-Ata, which postulated "Health for All" by the year 2000 (World Health Organization 1978).

With respect to the interaction among players in the health domain, we see a shift away from the idea that national governments are primarily responsible for their citizens' health, under the overall leadership and technical guidance of the WHO. Individuals across the globe, it is increasingly argued, should both contribute to the generation of health knowledge and have access to the fruits of that knowledge, independent of where they live. This thinking is evident in new concepts such as the "global public good," which postulates that knowledge about health must be generated and used in collaboration among diverse actors across national and cultural boundaries (Kaul and Faust 2001). An interesting institutional expression of this concept is the Institute for One World Health (iOWH), a "nonprofit drug company" founded in 2000 with the mission to develop new medicines for infectious diseases in developing countries (Hale, Woo, and Lipton 2005). The company's very name suggests that health is global; its institutional design (a company) suggests that it is part of the private sector, yet the label "nonprofit" suggests that its workings are a contribution to some form of greater public good.

We can make out the shape of an emerging global domain of public health policy in which four types of players interact. The first is the global patient, whose health is no longer solely determined by her allegiance to a particular nation-state, but by a variety of factors, including her own participation in the global domain. The second is a new global authority that governs the generation of knowledge and/or the delivery of health interventions through partnerships with multiple actors, including the global patient. The third player is the private sector, comprised of companies and nongovernmental organizations that contribute to global partnerships through the generation of knowledge, the contribution of financial means, or the provision of services. The fourth player is the nation-state, not about to disappear any time soon, which still exerts control over fundamental aspects of a patient's life— including the systems through which patients have access to health care. The state (or the government) now partners with the global authority, the private sector, and the patient in the global endeavor to improve health for all.

This image of a new global health domain raises fundamental questions for both policy makers and policy analysts. Far from erasing the previous system, the new global actors are entering a scene with existing players. They are changing the dynamics, gradually shifting the balance away from the WHO as the main supranational health body. In early 2008, an article in the *New York Times* charged the Bill and Melinda Gates Foundation with "wiping out the world health agency's policy making function" (McNeil Jr. 2008). Observations such as this raise important questions about who has a mandate to act on behalf of the public, about accountability and legitimacy, and about the respective authority of global, national, and local actors. As markets expand, GDPs grow, and patterns of health and disease change, who will be responsible for providing health care to patients throughout the world? And how can this best be done? In other words, how should we design a system of global health governance that is both fair and effective?

This book displays the emergence of the new global sector, with its rules, representations, and responsibilities, and elucidates how these are different from what was there before. It also investigates how this new level of policy making relates to the existing ones. Each chapter focuses on a different dimension of these processes of emergence and settling in. At the core of the book are four basic questions. First, how does an issue come to be regarded as "global"? Second, how do institutions emerge at the global level to address such issues? Third, what new rules, if any, do these new players introduce into the global domain, with regard to international action, nation-states, and their citizens? And, finally, how do these rules play out in practice in the interaction among various existing players? In order to address these questions, the study focuses on four entities: a globalizing sector (health), a global institution (the Global Fund), a global disease (HIV/AIDS), and a country (China).

The book draws on several fields of scholarly research, including most centrally the field of science and technology studies (STS). In the emerging global domain, which lacks obvious forms of political legitimation (such as representation of states or popular voting), knowledge production has become a principal pillar on which to establish legitimate political authority. Global actors need reliable knowledge as the basis for their presence and activity in the health domain (Long Martello and Jasanoff 2004). The STS idiom of co-production provides a useful way to conceptualize the connections among knowledge production, power, and institutions. Co-production refers to the process of natural and social orders being produced together (Jasanoff 2004). This framework enables us to study the means through which global and local actors mobilize knowledge to formulate and define a problem and its solution, and how new institutions and practices emerge in that process.

Co-production holds that moments of epistemic and normative emergence are related, indeed coupled in inseparable ways. Thus, the appearance of the "pandemic" HIV/AIDS accompanied the emergence of new forms of "global" governance of infectious diseases. Co-production happens via four interrelated pathways: the building of *representations, discourses, identities,* and *institutions* (Jasanoff 2004). In order for an issue to become the subject of public policy, there first needs to be a *representation,* a definition of what exactly the problem is and how it must be solved. This representation needs to become plausible to many. This in turn happens through *discourses* that transport the representation among individuals and enable it to become widely accepted. As part of these processes, social *identities* are created, as people come to see themselves in terms of the new representations and discourses. These can be new social groups that are the targets of policy (such as "single mothers," "people living with HIV/AIDS," or "injection drug users") or actors that assume well-defined roles in the policy-making process (such as "AIDS experts"). Finally, the problem is addressed by *institutions* whose design reflects the underlying representation of the problem. These four pathways of co-production happen anew for every policy issue that emerges and moves into the public domain.

Research in the co-productionist idiom can be divided into two main strands: the "constitutive" and the "interactionist" (Jasanoff 2004). The constitutive strand of co-production, rooted primarily in the work of Bruno Latour and the French school of actor-network theory, is mainly concerned with the role of representation in the construction of political authority (Jasanoff 2004, 25). Research in this strand focuses on the question of how new objects (ideas, technologies, or institutions) emerge and become stable parts of public life. In contrast, the interactionist strand of co-production, rooted mainly in the Edinburgh school of scientific sociology of knowledge, is concerned with the interaction between science and politics as two distinct spheres of authority (Jasanoff 2004). Research in this vein tends to focus on the ways in which scientific and technical controversies are resolved; the ways in which the products of science and technology are made intelligible and portable across cultural and other boundaries: and on the ways in which the processes of scientific knowledge production interact with their political and cultural environment (Jasanoff 2004, 39).

This work contributes to both strands of co-productionist research, each chapter focusing on a separate aspect of co-production. Chapters 2 and 3 are mainly accounts of the constitutive co-production of global health issues and global health institutions. Chapter 2 investigates how the different framings of tuberculosis, malaria, and HIV/AIDS—first as "biomedical," later as "social," and finally as "transnational" issues—relate to the ways in which they were addressed at the supranational level—first in specialized disease control programs, later through the strengthening of national primary health care infrastructure, and finally in "global public-private partnerships." Chapter 3 focuses on the co-production, at the turn of the millennium, of HIV/AIDS as a global health, human rights, and security issue and of the Global Fund as a global institution to address it. We witness the gradual evolution of the identity of a "global patient," whose health is no longer solely determined by nationality, and efforts to reach this patient through different forms of institutions. A view of the nature of disease as a multifactorial social, political, and economic issue is combined with a vision of global disease management as requiring the participation of multiple state and nonstate actors across local and global scales.

Chapters 4–6 are concerned with the Global Fund's institutional design and the ways in which it operates in the global domain. Chapter 4 focuses on the Global Fund as an institution, examining both constitutive and interactionist aspects of its existence. For example, what representational practices does the Global Fund employ to achieve its goals? How does it imagine the global domain and its players? And by what means can it get these players— governments, international agencies, civil society, and patients—to buy into its framings of health and illness? Similarly, how does the Fund shore up authority, create rules, and interact with existing players? How does the Fund imagine the boundary between science and politics? And how do these imaginations relate to the ways in which the Fund gains legitimacy and authority in the global domain?

Chapters 5 and 6 are devoted to the interaction between the Global Fund and one of its most important national grant recipients, China. Chapter 5 sets the background for this analysis, tracing the emergence of HIV/AIDS in China between 1985, when the first case of HIV was detected, and 2001, when China first started applying to the Global Fund for financial support of its national HIV/AIDS programs. The chapter focuses on processes of co-production at the national level. Upon detecting the first case of HIV/AIDS in China, the country's public health and scientific leadership presented it as a foreigner's disease. In order for it to become a national public health issue, HIV/AIDS first had to be understood as a Chinese problem. This required fundamental shifts not only in the way HIV/AIDS and sexuality were understood, but also in China's self-image—in the way people thought about Chinese culture, values, and human behavior in an era of deep-reaching socioeconomic change.

Chapter 6 focuses on the interaction between the Global Fund and China as an example of dealings between two different forms of governance: an emerging global (private) authority and an existing national government. Between 2002 and 2006, China's national HIV/AIDS policy agenda changed fundamentally to include all of the major tenets of the dominant international HIV/AIDS policy paradigm, including such controversial policies as providing sterile needles to injection drug users and fostering grassroots civil society. The chapter is an interactional co-productionist account: at its center are questions about the intelligibility and portability of products of science and knowledge from one context to another. Thus, how did the Global Fund's ideas about the way in which HIV/AIDS should be addressed become intelligible and applicable in China? And what role did the Global Fund's institutional design, with its reliance on stakeholder inclusion and scientific review, play in this process?

The study is at one level a case study investigating the coming into being of one of the most important and powerful recent institutional innovations in the emerging global health domain. This raises the question of what can be deduced from a single case. Are findings from this case generalizable, and if so in what sense? This question cannot be answered without touching on the Aristotelian question of whether any knowledge of the particular is possible or legitimate. How can we infer knowledge about the workings of the world from studying specific instances we select and observe? The historian of science John Forrester proposes that "reasoning in cases" is one valid style of reasoning alongside others, such as experimental exploration, postulation and deduction, and statistical analysis (Forrester 1996). Drawing on the history of psychoanalysis, on the historical sociology of the sciences, and on concepts of the individual in the human sciences, Forrester makes the argument that reasoning always happens from the particular to the particular. The invocation of any principle is always tied to and based on an example, a "prototype" (Forrester 1996). Cases then contain generalizable lessons because an implicit system of associations is embodied in them. This style of thinking, Forrester argues, also applies to the sciences of the state:

> We should be able to think about politics in this way [i.e., in cases], since we do it so easily. How often do political arguments, such as over the possibility of American intervention in Bosnia, revolve around selecting the right case to analogize from? Is Bosnia like Vietnam, a case of sacrificing American lives to influence the political and economic destiny of a far-off country? Or is it like

Europe in 1941, when a moral imperative that transcends any national self-interest can be invoked? . . . if you think that invoking principles will avoid this method of reasoning, a skeptic of the relevance of your principles will soon require you to make explicit the exemplar, the prototype, the analogue onto which the invocation of your principle is grafted.

(Forrester 1996, 21)

For the purpose of this study, then, one case is implicitly comparative. It compares empirical findings about the Global Fund and about global health governance to ideas about global governance that have been put out by the Global Fund and other actors. At another level, this work is also a study of the interaction between global and local levels in the emerging global domain.

This study draws on four categories of primary sources. First, in order to construct histories of global diseases, I searched the scientific literature for articles on HIV/AIDS, tuberculosis, and malaria between 1900 and 2007. I also "hand-searched" reports on scientific conferences, and medical and public health journals known for their coverage of matters of international health, including the *Bulletin of the World Health Organization, Science, Nature,* and *The Lancet.* A second major source consisted of newspaper articles. For Western sources on HIV/AIDS, tuberculosis, and malaria, I searched the *New York Times,* the *Washington Post,* and the *BBC.* In tracing the emergence of HIV/AIDS as a policy issue in China, I used Chinese and foreign media reporting on China (in English) during the period between 1980 and 2007, including the *China Daily,* the *People's Daily,* the *South China Morning Post,* and *Xinhua News Agency,* and the *New York Times, Agence France Presse,* and the *BBC.* Third, I used a variety of documents on the Global Fund itself. These include framework documents, by-laws, and internal sources, such as the applications submitted by China and other countries. I also searched the Global Fund Observer, a publication on the policy and strategic aspects of the Global Fund produced by a New York-based NGO called Aidspan (www.aidspan.org). Finally, my analysis is based on interviews with more than 40 individuals who played key roles in the different parts of this story. These include interviews with Global Fund officials at the organizations' headquarters in Geneva; Chinese government officials at the county, provincial, and central levels; representatives of international organizations that were members of the Chinese Country Coordinating Mechanism or the writing team for Global Fund applications; members of nongovernmental organizations in the Chinese HIV/AIDS sector; and representatives of foundations who worked in China.

The study yields three sets of theoretical and practical insights. First, it yields insights about the dynamics of co-production as it investigates fundamental questions about the emergence of new forms of governance. How do certain problems come to be understood as "global"? How do global institutions converge on certain ideas as constitutive of their mission and legitimacy? What is the relation between the global and the local, the uniform and the specific, particularly as regards the role of knowledge and expertise? How is a balance achieved between the global and the local? How much harmonization is desirable across localities, what kinds of harmonization can we hope for, and by what means should this harmonization be achieved?

Second, the study yields political insights about governance models for global institutions and standard setting in the global domain. How should a global entity in any sector balance between solutions framed at global and local scales? What kinds of governance structure should it adopt? How should it address questions of authority, legitimacy, and accountability, especially in its choice of process? With respect to standards and norms, the study critically examines several instances of settling for a new arrangement over an old one. For example, how did the international community move away from the dogmatic view that the provision of antiretroviral therapy to patients in developing countries was infeasible to the idea that all HIV/AIDS patients should have access to triple therapy? How did the international scientific community settle the ethical controversy about whether or not the use of placebo was justified in HIV/AIDS trials in the developing world? And how did China switch from one settlement about what kind of a problem HIV/AIDS is and what kind of solution it requires to a different settlement?

Finally, the study yields insights with respect to the institutional design and the work of the Global Fund. What has the Global Fund accomplished in the domain of public health policy? What kinds of powers does it have, and what are its practices for disseminating a global perspective? To the extent that these erase local particularities, are they desirable? What are the features of institutional design that have made the Global Fund successful, in its own or other terms? And finally, what can we learn from the Global Fund's example as other global issues emerge in the health domain and in other domains?

Policy makers should find these insights useful. The Global Fund is arguably the most powerful and innovative of the recently founded public-private partnerships. Since its inception in 2002, it has disbursed more than eight billion USD for programs in over 130 developing countries (The Global Fund to Fight Aids, Tuberculosis and Malaria 2003). Its emergence has been rapid and remarkable. Designed to circumvent major flaws in bilateral and multilateral development aid including "donor drivenness" and a perceived failure to create sustainable results (Richards 2001; Yamey and Rankin 2002), the Global Fund has been hailed as a new model of governance (Richards 2001; Poku 2002). Its workings are thought to have important implications for financial aid in sectors other than health, for example, the provision of education in the developing world (Jamison and Radelet 2005).

Given the amounts of resources and large hopes invested in the Fund, its every move is under intense scrutiny. Important questions are at stake. Is the Global Fund really a new, better kind of solution to problems of supranational governance? Have we finally found a way to design institutions that can deliver sustainable results across national and cultural boundaries in response to some of the most pressing challenges to human well-being? In addressing these questions, many focus on quantitative measures of the Global Fund's success. Some ask, for example, how many people have gained access to treatment as a consequence of the Fund's work since 2002, and where this puts us with respect to targets for combating the three diseases as specified in the millennium goals (Komatsu et al. 2007). Others focus on the question of how developing countries, given their weak health infrastructures, can absorb the large amount of funding that has so suddenly become available through this new organization (Lu et al. 2006). Yet others examine operational indicators of the Fund's work, such as the correlation between program evaluation scores and program characteristics in Fund-financed programs (Radelet and Siddiqi 2007).

These questions are important, and so are their answers for the continued evolution and success of the Global Fund. However, equally, if not more, important are qualitative aspects of the Fund's influence. How does this new organization work, and how does its vision of global health policy making play out in reality? How does it interact with governments? What are its effects on standards and norms in the health domain? Is it able to induce governments to engage civil society and patients in a new kind of global partnership to combat HIV/AIDS, tuberculosis, and malaria? And what do the details of this cooperation look like? Ultimately, in-depth knowledge of how the Global Fund interacts with recipient countries and with other actors in the health domain will be a crucial element in our understanding of the successes and (potential) failures of this bold new model. After all, the Fund's emergence and evolution have not just meant the disbursement of money to more than 130 countries. It also implies the rapid rolling out of a new form of political and policy engagement between a global authority and local actors. The Global Fund is an agent of epistemic, political, and social change, at the same time that it is also a development aid organization. The details of its interactions with states and civil societies are little understood. It is here that this study hopes to make its most salient contribution.

CHAPTER 2

Public Health in the Twenty-First Century: Beyond the Multilateral Institutions

This chapter discusses the processes through which a health issue comes to be understood as global. It traces the evolution of international institutional responses to three health issues that have attained global status—tuberculosis, malaria, and HIV/AIDS—since their emergence. Several factors play a role in determining the global status of these health issues. These factors include the severity and distribution of the disease, the rapidity of its spread, the societal groups it affects, and the availability of a cure. Once a combination of these factors is present, global status can be conferred on the basis of three categories that are seen as transcending national boundaries—"biomedicine," "human rights," and "transnational nature." Over time, these three framings shaped, often in competition among each other, varying approaches to the control of tuberculosis, malaria, and HIV/AIDS. In the 1980s and 1990s, all three were seen as intimately intertwined with globalization. The idea that partnerships between governments, intergovernmental organizations, companies, and civil society were the best ways to address these health issues became dominant in the public health community.

Until the 1980s, biomedicine and human rights were the two main frameworks that served as the basis for the claim that a health issue was "global." When antibiotics and vaccines became available, tuberculosis and malaria became represented as solvable *biomedical problems*. According to this view, the afflicted patient becomes a citizen in a treatment regime that is seen as easily traveling across national and cultural boundaries. Correspondingly, institutional responses focus on the goal of delivering technologies to affected individuals through specialized disease control structures. In contrast, the framing of health and disease as a *human rights issue* puts at the center of its concern the healthy individual that needs protection from a variety of illnesses throughout lifetime. Access to primary health care services is conceptualized as a right that transcends culture and nationality. Institutional responses in this framework focus mainly on the construction of health care infrastructure. Over time, the two competing framings of "disease as biomedicine" and of "health as a human right" played a role in the institutionalization of all three diseases. Both regard the nation-state as the principal provider of health care to its citizens. By the end of the 1980s, the WHO's efforts – under both of these paradigms – had come to be regarded insufficient in their ability to address local diversity and effectively reach the grassroots levels.

In the 1990s, another form of global status emerged. All three diseases became seen as intimately intertwined with globalization, or as *transnational*. In this model, the responsibility for providing health care is no longer solely assigned to governments, but it rests on partnerships of state and non-state actors. The patient becomes an *agent* in a system in which multiple actors are connected across local, national, and supranational scales. The concept of partnerships is thus conceived of as an institutional structure that encompasses both the "transnational" and the "local."

The Co-production of Public Health Issues and Public Health Institutions

Public health is a field of political struggle that intrinsically centers on the tension between individual liberties and the government's right and obligation to protect the health of the community. When a disease or health hazard appears, three fundamental issues must be negotiated before the hazard can become the subject of public health policy. First, whose problem is it? Second, how should the problem be brought under control? And third, whose responsibility is it to do so? If the issue is recognized as a disease or health hazard that affects the public, it can then move from the domain of individual responsibility into the domain of collective responsibility. Finally, authorities come to deal with it. The need to protect healthy individuals from the threat of disease justifies public action.

In the process, a boundary is created between those affected and those who are not affected by the disease (I will call this an "*us/other boundary*"). Intimately intertwined with this is the question of how to deal with the diseased "other." Should that "other" be regarded as a potential threat, even a transgressor, and dealt with using law enforcement techniques? Alternatively, should the "other" be seen as a patient, as someone to empathize with? These competing framings are illustrated in the 2007 international public health scandal over the question of how to treat a U.S. citizen who had apparently traveled despite warnings from state health officials that he was infected with tuberculosis—there was an intense debate over whether he had acted irresponsibly and whether or not the authorities should have forcibly restricted his movement (Schwartz 2007).[1] This illustrates how, in one single case, the two framings can compete, as the representatives of the state are caught between two responsibilities: that of supporting a citizen with a health problem and of guaranteeing that the same individual does not endanger public safety through a potential spread of his or her infection.

The STS idiom of *co-production* helps us to understand the processes through which an issue becomes the subject of public policy. As discussed in Chapter 1, co-production happens through the making of *representations, discourses, identities,* and *institutions* (Jasanoff 2004, 39), which happen anew for every policy issue that emerges in a society. As this chapter will illustrate, the processes of co-production not only operate at the national level, but can also be equally observed at the global level. For a public health issue to be regarded as "global," a perceived mechanism must exist by which the issue or some of its aspects travel across national boundaries such that the creation and involvement of supranational actors are required to address it. Before I discuss the specific cases of tuberculosis, malaria, and HIV/AIDS, I will address a number of general trends that affected the way these diseases became understood.

International Health Cooperation in the Twentieth Century

Until the 1980s, two mechanisms emerged by which health and disease could become regarded as global. The first is biomedicine. Biomedical representations of a disease generally serve the purpose of identifying clear targets and demonstrable results. At the center of this paradigm is the *afflicted individual* that needs protection from a *specific condition.* Biomedicine is then seen as an equalizing force yielding technologies that are effective regardless of the social, cultural, or national context in which they are used—its concepts universalize the status of the patient and decouple it from nationality or culture.

Based on this view of science and medicine, the increasing availability of antibiotics and vaccines in the 1930s and 1940s generated great enthusiasm among international public health experts. Many infectious diseases suddenly appeared preventable and/or curable, and public health suddenly seemed to possess the power to eliminate tremendous levels of suffering and death all over the world. Freedom from TB, malaria, and other infections, it was hoped, would now be within everyone's reach (Maher and Nunn 1998; Raviglione and Pio 2002). This meant a redefinition of the purpose of international health cooperation, a shift away from Westphalian principles, which had been designed to enable disease control for the improvement of dealings between sovereign states, toward the principle of furthering not just disease control but also the provision of health care to all patients suffering from a given illness.

In the first half of the twentieth century, the WHO built *vertical* disease control programs (Raviglione and Pio 2002). These programs were designed to deliver newly available drugs and vaccines for a range of infectious diseases—including malaria, tuberculosis, and leprosy—in a "single-purpose machinery, independent of both the general health infrastructure and the structure of other vertical programmes" (Raviglione and Pio 2002). Vertical programs were designed and set up to run separately from national health infrastructure. They reflect the view that specialized expertise and focus were needed to make a dent in these infectious diseases, which were best delivered through a targeted, centralized structure.

Throughout the twentieth century, these vertical approaches competed with *horizontal* approaches, which sought to make primary health care available to all humans. At the center of this paradigm, which was also initiated by the WHO, was the *healthy individual* in need of protection from a range of diseases throughout lifetime. This required not single-focus interventions, but rather a complicated system of prevention, treatment, and care. Under the rubric "Health for All by 2000," the WHO's 1978 Alma-Ata Declaration, defining health as a "state of complete wellbeing" (rather than as the absence of disease), affirmed humanity's right to basic health care services (World Health Organization 1978). The idea that individuals have a "right to health" universalizes the status of the patient and decouples it from nationality and culture. In analogy to the idea that all patients with a given disease should receive treatment, the construction of a right to primary health care is a departure from the Westphalian principle of noninterference. Yet similar to the vertical approach, the horizontal model of supranational public health cooperation also conceptualized the nation-state as the main provider of health care.[2] In both cases, the WHO, through its legitimacy as a UN organization, provides advice and technical assistance to governments of sovereign states to improve the health of their populations.

(Re)Defining Health and Disease

In the second half of the twentieth century, that idea changed radically, when health and disease were fundamentally reconceptualized. The existing *representation* of health and disease changed in four major ways. First, the biomedical view of health and disease was increasingly challenged. Today, most health issues are conceptualized as complex and cross-cutting economic, social, behavioral, and political issues that require broad approaches and thinking beyond biomedicine. This has been true for infectious diseases for a while, as the remainder of the chapter will show, and increasingly also for noncommunicable diseases. However, and more surprisingly, the same thinking is being applied more and more frequently even to problems that were not commonly seen as belonging to the core of international public health policy—the most recent, prominent examples of such issues include smoking and tobacco-related illnesses (Davis et al. 2007; Ebrahim et al. 2007), obesity (Chopra, Galbraith, and Darnton-Hill 2002; Chopra and Darnton-Hill 2004; Ebrahim et al. 2007), road traffic accidents (Mathers and Loncar 2006), and violence (Rutherford et al. 2007). WHO's Framework Convention on Tobacco Control (FCTC) is an example of emerging global health governance to address one of these new types of public health issues (tobacco-related illnesses) (Satcher 1999).

Second, the representation of the way health and disease are distributed in the world has changed. The concept of the *epidemiological transition,* originally proposed by Omran in 1971 (Omran 2005), gained currency. His proposition that with rising economic status the epidemiological profile of the diseases affecting populations in developing countries would also change, with an expected rise in noncommunicable diseases like cardiovascular problems, cancer, and tobacco-related illnesses, has come to be widely accepted and used (see, for example, Yusuf, Ounpuu, and Anand 2002; Kanavos 2006; Davis et al. 2007). The 1996 Global Burden of Disease Study, carried out by health and development experts at Harvard, at the WHO, and at the World Bank, marked the beginning of systematic cross-national assessment of health and disease by the UN bodies and placed noncommunicable diseases among the top health problems in the world (Murray and Lopez 1990; Lopez et al. 2006; Mathers and Loncar 2006).

Third, the relation between health and economic development has been reconceptualized. Health is increasingly seen as a means rather than purely as a consequence of production. Consequently, health policy was increasingly presented as a pillar of successful economic policy rather than as its automatic by-product. The 1993 World Bank Report entitled "Investing in Health" made the argument that developing countries need to actively invest in improving the health of their populations as part of their economic development (World Bank 1993). Later efforts of WHO under Gro Harlem Brundtland worked to strengthen and refine the evidence for this argument (Commission on Macroeconomics and Health 2001). The increased importance that health care has since been given on the development agenda is also illustrated by the fact that 4 of the 10 Millennium Development Goals are related to health.[3]

Disease are increasingly understood as transnational. The spread of diseases is perceived as more threatening in a world that is becoming more and more connected. In the 1980s, the rapid spread of HIV/AIDS epidemic throughout the globe forcefully drove home the point that infectious diseases do not stop at national boundaries. Antibiotic-resistant malaria and tuberculosis, SARS, anthrax, and bird flu have since followed to strengthen that conviction. Fittingly, SARS has been labeled the "first post-Westphalian pathogen" (Fidler 2003).

Not only infections but also behavior is increasingly conceptualized as transcending national boundaries. Recently, the argument has been made that "behavioral risks" that lead to health problems such as obesity and tobacco-related illnesses are in the process of becoming global (Ebrahim et al. 2007). Similarly, with scientists applying new approaches like social network theory to the problem of obesity (Christakis and Fowler 2007), being overweight has been conceptualized as sharing aspects of contagion ("Obesity 'contagious', experts say" 2007). The fast food and tobacco industries are accused of causing or at least substantially contributing to the spread of these problems (Chopra and Darnton-Hill 2004). New forms of international treaties and regulations are being instituted at the supranational level, such as the FCTC (Satcher 1999), which need to reflect the multifactorial, cross-disciplinary nature of the problems they have been designed to tackle.

(Re)Defining Responsibility

Co-production allows us to see that the changes in the way health and disease are represented have come hand-in-hand with propositions to change the ways in which we address them. When international health cooperation started in the mid-nineteenth century, it came out of the experience of two cholera epidemics in 1830 and 1847, which had killed tens of thousands of Europeans (McCarthy 2002). It had the primary goal of containing the spread of infectious diseases so that travel and trade between sovereign states would be enhanced (McCarthy 2002; Fidler 2003). No assumption was made that international institutions would in any way interfere with the internal workings of sovereign states. As I argued earlier, the WHO's initiation of vertical and horizontal programs represents a step away from that original concept. Both the biomedical framework and the human rights view of health assume that governments will work to improve their populations' health under the leadership of the WHO.

In the latter half of the 1990s, a fundamental change occurred, a shift away from the UN-centered—and, in the case of health, WHO-centered—landscape to a landscape in which both state and nonstate actors play a role.

Health, environmental protection, and security have increasingly become conceptualized as "global public goods" (Reinicke 1997) that require the participation of multiple actors in the production and distribution to humanity independent of national boundaries. In the health sector, more than 100 new "global public—private partnerships" have emerged in the 1990s (World Health Organization 2001; Widdus 2005). They differ substantially in terms of size, mission, activities, and players involved (Widdus 2001). Some focus on the production of new knowledge and tools for combating diseases that mainly affect patients in developing countries, like the Medicines for Malaria Venture and the Global Alliance for TB Drug Development; others aim to make prevention and treatment available to patients in developing countries, like the Global Fund to Fight Aids, Tuberculosis and Malaria or the partnership between the pharmaceutical company Merck, the UN agencies, and developing country governments, which has made a cure for river blindness available for millions of patients (Thylefors, Alleman, and Twum-Danso 2008). The common thing between them is that they draw on public and private sector partners and that they are not affiliated with governmental or intergovernmental agencies.

This trend toward partnerships is new. Until the late 1970s, there was very little cooperation between private and public sectors in the area of international development (Buse and Walt 2000a, 2000b). A variety of explanations can be given for this change. Thus, some explain it to be the result of a change in the way the state's role in the provision of public services is conceptualized, with an increasing emphasis on engaging markets and increasing efficiency (Poku and Whiteside 2002). Others see a general loss of faith in the capability of national governments and the multilateral institutions to solve the problems commonly associated with globalization at the origin of recent calls for "post-Westphalian public health governance" (Aginam 2006).

However, the overall significance of the trends I have outlined in the preceding section, including that toward "partnerships," is the fact that they imply a fundamental reassignment of responsibilities, at least in theory, away from the nation-states and multilateral institutions onto a larger, more diverse array of players. The argument is that if a disease is not simply biomedical but rather a matter of society, economics, culture, and behavior, and if it does not halt on national borders, then surely governments and the multilateral institutions can no longer be expected to provide solutions on their own. At stake is a fundamental question: as markets expand, GDPs grow, and patterns of health and disease change, who has the responsibility for providing health care in developing countries?

The WHO has been an active driver of this evolution. As the following chapters will show, Gro Harlem Brundtland, who took office as WHO's

Director-General in 1998, restructured large parts of WHO's work on tuberculosis and malaria from WHO-driven efforts to more loose, cross-sectoral partnerships. Her speech, at the 55th World Health Assembly in 2002, emphasizing the need for this new governance model, expresses the notion that in today's globalizing world, effective policy can no longer come from single bodies or institutions acting according to Westphalian principles:

> In a world filled with complex health problems, the WHO can not solve them alone. Governments cannot solve them all. Non-governmental organizations, the private sector and foundations cannot solve them. Only the new partnerships can make a difference and the evidence shows we are. Whether we like it or not, we are dependent on the partners, the resources and the energy necessary for at least a 30-fold scale-up in an effort—to bridge the gap and achieve health for all.
>
> (Brundtland 2002)

Two prominent examples of the new approach she introduced to international public health are the multilateral partnerships "Stop TB" and "Roll Back Malaria."

In some instances, "post-Westphalian" approaches taken by the WHO have triggered a direct reaction from its member states. In 2001, the World Health Report published a ranking of 191 national health systems according to various indicators of the overall quality of their performance (World Health Organization 2000b), which generated a lot of attention in both scientific and nonscientific press. A discussion quickly emerged on whether or not the methodology of the study had been adept to adequately reflect what it purported to measure and to what extend that was even measurable (Gravelle et al. 2003; Hollingsworth and Wildman 2003; Nolte and McKee 2003). These controversies illustrate the friction that can occur with the change in role that the WHO was effectively assuming with the publishing of this assessment—that of a public arbitrator of the quality of national governments' efforts to protect the health of their citizens, rather than that of a pure knowledge broker and technical advisor to support whichever strategies its member states chose to pursue.

Tuberculosis: From Sanatoria to "Stop TB"

Humanity has struggled with tuberculosis for thousands of years. It is believed to have been the leading cause of death in the history of the industrialized world (Bloom and Murray 1992). The disease is present in every region of the world and affects adults and children, men and women, alike. Over time, it has come to be seen as intimately intertwined with poverty and social inequality.

International approaches to tuberculosis gained momentum when antibiotics became available. Over the course of the twentieth century, the international tuberculosis control paradigm shifted back and forth between *vertical* and *horizontal* approaches; neither was regarded as particularly successful, as both were seen as unable to adequately address the specificities of varying local context. As the following sections will show, the representation of tuberculosis shifted over time, from a biomedical problem requiring antibiotics and vaccines to a multifactorial problem requiring an organizational solution to the intricacies of large-scale distribution of medical treatment.

Sanatoria Versus Primary Health Care

TB first attained priority status on the international public health agenda in the 1940s, when streptomycin, the first antibiotic shown to be effective against it, was discovered. As Raviglione and Pio discuss in their excellent review of the history of tuberculosis control in the second half of the twentieth century, a centralized TB unit was established at the WHO in 1947—the increasing availability after World War II of chemotherapy against infectious diseases and of insecticides for vector elimination had triggered the creation of so-called *vertical programs* within the WHO, each reaching from the center to the periphery, but with little direct connection to existing national health structures or to other WHO disease control programs (Raviglione and Pio 2002). At the time, TB was the leading infectious killer in developing countries, and it was hoped that the combination of antibiotics and mass vaccination with the BCG vaccine could make prevention and treatment available to many (Maher and Nunn 1998; Raviglione and Pio 2002).

The WHO's vertical control programs were successful in industrialized countries. Starting in the 1950s, the discovery and use of other TB drugs including isoniazid in 1952, p-amino salicylic acid, and pyrazinamide led to a continued reduction of TB mortality in the industrialized world (Bloom and Murray 1992). By that time, TB could be prevented with isoniazid in people who were exposed to it; infected individuals could be rendered noncontagious with combinations of available antibiotics and then cured (Verhoef 1994). The combination of case-finding and treatment of infectious cases in specialized TB sanatoria with mass vaccination at birth led to declines in tuberculosis rates by 10–15 percent annually, an important improvement compared to the earlier 4–5 percent that sanatoria alone had been able to achieve (Kochi 1991). BCG became the most widely used vaccine in the world (Bloom and Murray 1992).[4]

These successes, however, could not be replicated in developing countries. According to Raviglione and Pio, it became clear in the late 1950s that the strategy was not working in the same way. The reasons for this were seen in the difficulties of implementing vertical strategies in the developing country context—thus, they argue that the detection strategies used by industrialized countries to quickly identify TB cases in large numbers did not work in the same way in developing countries, that vertical TB control programs could not easily be extended to whole countries due to their specialized structure, and that the cost of the programs was too high, especially when it came to the deployment of newer TB drugs like rifampicin and pyrazinamide, which were largely unaffordable in resource-poor settings (Raviglione and Pio 2002). The vertical structure, it seems, did not lend itself to responding to local specificities. TB continued to be the leading killer among infectious diseases in developing countries (Bloom and Murray 1992).

In the early 1960s, this changed, after public health evidence from the developing country context was mobilized to challenge the vertical approach. The scientific basis for this change came at least in part out of public health work in Asia. In this region of the world, tuberculosis was treated in the ambulatory setting out of sheer necessity—infection rates were high, and hospital beds could not be made available to all infected patients (see Fox 1958, 1962; Bayer and Wilkinson 1995). The Tuberculosis Chemotherapy Centre in Madras, a research institution supported by the Indian government, the WHO, and the British Medical Research Council, did important work in the 1950 and 1960s, showing that TB control was feasible without sanatoria and that most infections could be successfully detected through screening programs in general health clinics (Banerji 1965; Kamat et al. 1966). Based on this collaboration between local and international tuberculosis experts, it was argued that TB control did not need vertical programs but could be done in general health clinics (Kamat et al. 1966).

During the period 1964–1976, the vertical approach to TB was substituted with a horizontal one. Specialized tuberculosis programs were integrated into the national health infrastructure, and TB clinics changed to general health facilities (Raviglione and Pio 2002). A central element of the new strategy was the supervised ambulatory treatment of TB patients, based on experience from other infectious diseases (Raviglione and Pio 2002). Tuberculosis was now being presented as a problem of "social planning" (Banerji 1965), an "organizational exercise in the provision of ambulatory care" (Maher and Nunn 1998). The efforts were reinforced by the growing influence of the primary health care movement as described in the declaration of Alma-Ata in 1978 (World Health Organization 1978) and continued throughout the 1970s as part of an ongoing "health sector reform," comprised of the "decentralization of authority," the "managerial integration of programs," and "public consultation" (Raviglione and Pio 2002).

But the outcome of the horizontal strategy was no more encouraging than the vertical approach had been. The mortality toll that tuberculosis was taking on developing country populations could not be substantially reduced—rates of decline were less than 50 percent of those observed in industrialized countries (Raviglione and Pio 2002). The methods of TB case management—detection, diagnosis, and chemotherapy—were apparently hard to apply in developing countries (see, for example, Pio 1989). In 1976, Styblo et al. showed that while the BCG vaccine effectively prevents childhood tuberculosis, it does not break the chain of TB transmission on the population level and therefore does not show the epidemiological effects that had been hoped for (Styblo and Meijer 1976). This further weakened the argument of those who held that humanity had the tools necessary to stop TB.

By the early 1980s, the public health community's attention for TB gradually started to lessen. Raviglione and Pio note a decrease in the activity of the key actors that had spearheaded international scientific and public health work in the TB control domain: the Bulletin of the WHO ceased publishing its special issues on TB; the International Tuberculosis Conference halved its frequency to once every four years; in 1985, the British Medical Council closed its TB unit, which had been key in driving scientific refinements in TB control methodology; and even the WHO apparently downsized and restructured its investments—by 1989, WHO Tuberculosis staff had been reduced to two experts, and the formerly separate TB structures in WHO's regional offices had been integrated into existing infectious diseases entities (Raviglione and Pio 2002). The realization that effective TB control or even eradication were not within reach in developing countries, combined with the absence of an acute TB threat in the industrialized world, had changed the perception of TB as a scourge that could be tackled if only the international community devoted enough attention to it.

DOTS: The Organizational Approach to TB

In the mid-1980s, TB reemerged in the industrialized world. In 1984, U.S. TB notification rates went up instead of falling and increased throughout the 1980s and 1990s (Bloom and Murray 1992; Neville et al. 1993), giving rise to what was termed the "U-shaped curve of concern" (Reichman 1991). Similar rises were observed in Western Europe (Raviglione et al. 1993) and in the former Soviet Union (Raviglione 2003). In the United States, several factors were thought to be responsible for this trend: the rise in HIV and in urban poverty (Brudney and Dobkin 1991) and increasing levels of migration

(McKenna, McCray, and Onorato 1995). Tuberculosis in the United States came to be understood as interconnected with tuberculosis elsewhere. One observer noted: "it will be difficult to eliminate tuberculosis without better efforts to prevent and control it among immigrants and greater efforts to control it in the countries from which they come" (McKenna, McCray, and Onorato 1995).

This perception of interconnectedness, together with the resurgence of incidence and prevalence, put TB back in the international spotlight. In 1989/1990, WHO undertook a special study to assess the global burden of TB (Kochi 1991; Sudre, Tendam, and Kochi 1992). The study estimated that one-third of the world's population was infected with TB and that in 1990, 2.9 million died of the disease (Sudre, Tendam, and Kochi 1992). In the decade preceding 1990, 2.5–3.2 million cases of TB had been reported to the WHO annually, most of them in Asia (Sudre, Tendam, and Kochi 1992). It was estimated that in developing countries, more than 80 percent of tuberculosis incidence and mortality occurred in TB-affected individuals in the prime of their productivity, a pattern very different to that observed in industrialized countries, where tuberculosis mainly occurred in the elderly, and usually as a consequence of reactivation of an existing dormant infection (Kochi 1991).

Based on this report, Arata Kochi, head of the new WHO Global Program on Tuberculosis (GPT), presented a new global control strategy that later became famous as "DOTS," or Directly Observed Treatment Short-Course (Kochi 1991). Still at the center of this strategy was the direct supervision of patient medication. However, it now came with a shortened course of TB chemotherapy, which represented a substantial simplification of the treatment regimen. Again, the scientific evidence for the strategy came from research conducted in developing countries. Based on a number of national TB programs run at the International Union Against Tuberculosis and Lung Disease (IUATLD), a scientist named Karel Styblo had reported cure rates of 80 percent in Tanzania, Malawi, and Mozambique with a directly supervised, short-course drug regimen (Raviglione and Pio 2002). The method was not entirely new (it was taken from a 1973 report of the WHO Expert Committee on TB), but Styblo had refined it with a more rigorous way of analyzing program outcomes (cohort analysis) (Raviglione 2003).

DOTS was believed to be able to better address earlier failures to address local-level specificities. It is worth taking a look at the reasons that were given for these failures. Arata Kochi's account from the time foreshadow many of the arguments that dominated the discussion, about a decade later, about whether or not antiretroviral therapy should be provided to patients in developing countries:

"1. Technical policies are largely concentrated on 'what should and could be done' in relatively well-developed health service systems . . . and often lack the component of 'how to do it' under different settings. 2. Some of the intervention technologies, which are effective, simple and affordable in well-developed health service systems, are not necessarily effective, simple and affordable in poorly developed health service systems. 3. Some of the technical policies appear to have been taken as dogma . . . so that there has been a tendency to discourage result-orientated and local innovative approaches".

(Kochi 1991)

In Kochi's argument, an inability or unwillingness to adapt to local circumstances and to foster local ideas, knowledge, and innovation was at the heart of pre-DOTS failures.

DOTS quickly came to be seen as a breakthrough in international health. Kochi's 1990 publication (Kochi 1991) had generated attention in the public health community (Sbarbaro 2001). Through DOTS, WHO wanted to achieve an overall reduction in the annual death rate from TB by 40 percent and "an 85 percent cure rate of all sputum-positive patients under treatment" as well as "70 percent case detection" by the year 2000 (Kochi 1991). These targets were adopted in a resolution of the 44th World Health Assembly in 1991 (Raviglione 2003). The enthusiasm continued throughout the 1990s. The 1993 World Bank Report declared tuberculosis control "one of the most cost-effective of all interventions" in primary health care of the time (World Bank 1993). In 1997, WHO's Director-General referred to DOTS as the leading advancement in international health of the decade (Smith 1999).

Yet DOTS was not able to stem the tide, either. HIV continued to play a major role in the renewed spread of tuberculosis worldwide (World Health Organization 1989).[5] And in the early 1990s, outbreaks of multi-drug-resistant tuberculosis (MDR-TB) occurred in the United States (Centers for Disease Control and Prevention 1990a, 1990b) and some locations in Europe (Iseman 1998).[6] A 1991 TB report by the United States Centers for Disease Control found that 13.3 percent of TB cases were resistant to at least one anti-tuberculosis drug, and 3 percent were resistant to both isoniazid and rifampicin (Villarino, Geiter, and Simone 1992). Some called MDR-TB the "third epidemic" (with HIV being the first and HIV/TB the second) (Neville et al. 1993), and experts warned that unless the spread was halted, the world was going to be left with old-fashioned tools common before the advent of antibiotics—as one commentator put it, describing that scenario, "it is back to sanatoria, surgery and cod-liver oil" (Veen 1995).

In 1993, the WHO declared TB a global emergency ("Tuberculosis: a global emergency" 1993). But while the United States successfully contained its TB resurgence—albeit at a cost exceeding US$ 400 million in New York

City alone (Frieden et al. 1995)—there was, at first, no agreement about what was to be done about rising MDR-TB rates in developing countries.[7] MDR-TB warnings from developing countries had first appeared in the mid-1980s (Iseman 1985). For example, reports from Peru's national TB program showed low treatment success rates (Hopewell et al. 1984) and later primary drug resistance rates of 25 percent (Hopewell et al. 1985), even though the program had been considered successful (Farmer et al. 1998).

However, there was disagreement over whether MDR-TB was really a global problem. Some argued, notwithstanding its presence in a large number of countries, that the disease was really focal in nature, with local, circumscribed outbreaks in Nepal (48 percent), the Indian State of Gujarat (33.8 percent), New York City (30.1 percent), Bolivia (15.3 percent), and Korea (14.5 percent) (Cohn, Bustreo, and Raviglione 1997). Others, citing evidence from a joint survey by the WHO and the IUATLD showing that MDR-TB was present in all of the 35 countries and regions that had been investigated, argued it was global in nature (Pablos-Mendez et al. 1998).

Again, the arguments parallel those of the controversies regarding the provision of antiretroviral treatment. Was treating MDR-TB all over the world the right approach? Was it feasible? In 1998, Harvard's Paul Farmer and a group of colleagues made the argument that specialized treatment of MDR-TB needed to be made available to all affected patients, pointing to the "transnational nature of the modern TB pandemic" (Farmer et al. 1998). Critical voices held that global expansion of treatment for MDR-TB was too complicated and simply not cost-effective (Espinal et al. 1999; Smith 1999) and warned that focusing on MDR-TB would draw away resources from treating patients with nonresistant TB (Smith 1999).

In 1998 the WHO finally issued the *DOTS Plus* strategy, adding specialized treatment facilities and programs for MDR-TB to the existing DOTS programs (Iseman 1998). To address the cost of second-line TB drugs, one of the major constraints to MDR-TB control, the WHO established the Green Light Committee Initiative (GLC) with the aim to develop solutions (such as special price arrangements with pharmaceutical companies) that would lower the prices of certain TB drugs (Raviglione and Pio 2002).

"Stop TB": The Era of Partnerships

By the late 1990s, it had become clear that DOTS could not reach the needed coverage. Raviglione and Pio argue that the main challenge was not the *adoption* of DOTS at the national level but the *scaling up* of functioning pilot programs to the whole country, especially in the 22 countries that had 80 percent of the global TB burden (Raviglione and Pio 2002; Raviglione

2003)—even after its adoption in 127 countries by 1999 (as a consequence of increased funding[8]), DOTS reached only about 20 percent of all TB cases at that time (Raviglione and Pio 2002). Clearly, adoption at the government level did not automatically guarantee success at the local level.

WHO's new Director-General Gro Harlem Brundtland convened the "Ad-hoc Committee on the TB Epidemic" in March 1998 in London to discuss the world TB situation (World Health Organization 1998b). The committee issued an influential report that noted the lack of progress, identified major constraints to the success of DOTS,[9] and recommended a more comprehensive and multisectoral approach to addressing it (World Health Organization 1998b, 2006; Raviglione 2003).

Under Brundtland's leadership, the TB landscape was fundamentally restructured at the end of the 1990s. In 1998, the Global TB Program was closed and replaced with the *Stop TB Partnership* (Raviglione 2003). It was formed as a public–private partnership, a coalition of governments, nongovernmental organizations, donors, and other TB-related organizations. Some even argued it had "evolved from a partnership of international organizations into a global social movement" (Lee, Loevinsohn, and Kumaresan 2002).

As was the case for earlier approaches, the aim of the new program was to eliminate tuberculosis as a public health problem, with the mission to ensure that every TB patient gained access to effective diagnosis, treatment, and cure (Kumaresan et al. 2004).[10] However, in addition to DOTS expansion through national health structures, it previewed the construction of three new global research and development partnerships for new TB tools (drugs, diagnostics, and vaccines).[11,12] One of these initiatives, the Global Alliance on TB Drug Development, has created a tuberculosis drug discovery program ("Tuberculosis: GlaxoSmithKline and TB Alliance Renew Tuberculosis Drug Discovery Program" 2008).

Thus, the representation of tuberculosis had shifted over time, and with it, the approaches proposed to address the disease. First, it was seen as a biomedical problem that could be tackled with defined, globally applicable tools, like vaccines and antibiotics; that representation changed later to one that presented tuberculosis as a matter of the right organizational skills and systems, which the state, with the support from WHO's programs, could deploy, together with biomedical tools, to reach patients in its realm; finally, after efforts to control tuberculosis in the developing world had failed and MDR-TB had appeared and risen instead, tuberculosis came to be represented as a transnational problem that governments and the WHO could no longer solve on their own. For example, the high cost of certain tuberculosis drugs, which had been seen to be governed by the markets and thus as lying outside of the direct public health "jurisdiction" of national governments and the WHO, was included in the problem definition. In line with this view, a partnership was created that brought together a wide variety of state and nonstate actors, including the private sector.

Malaria: From Control to Eradication and Back

Forty percent of all human beings live with a continuous threat of contracting malaria, a diseases thought to kill about 1 million people and to cause 500 million severe infections annually (World Health Organization 2007). As is the case for tuberculosis, malaria has been present for thousands of years. Malaria is different from tuberculosis in that it has distinct environmental and geographic components. Malaria is a classic "tropical disease," and its agent, a parasite called *plasmodium,* is transmitted through the anopheles mosquito, which needs a certain climate to thrive, limiting the distribution of malaria to hot and humid geographic zones. The way malaria afflicts human beings is intimately connected with the patients' previous immunological exposure to it. Its fatal form disproportionately affects small children who have not been exposed to the disease (or, by the same token, travelers to malarious regions), whereas adults in endemic reasons usually experience comparatively milder symptoms due to their having acquired partial immunity (Carter and Mendis 2002).[13,14]

As the following section will show, institutional approaches to malaria have cycled back and forth between efforts at control and attempts at eradication. Before the discovery of the malaria cycle in 1880, by French military physician Alphonse Laveran, public health intervention against malaria consisted mainly of swamp draining. The discovery of the cycle put a number of concrete targets within reach: the adult mosquito in the environment; its larvae, which dwell in standing waters; and the parasite *plasmodium* in its different developmental stages inside the human body. The newly gained knowledge of the different components of this system suggested to many that it could be disrupted. Italian malariologist Battista Grassi famously referred to malaria as a "giant with feet of clay" (Coluzzi 1999), suggesting that if humanity was able to successfully target a fragile spot in this cycle, malaria would crumble at once.

Over time, this representation of malaria as a biomedical problem with defined technical solutions was replaced by an image of malaria as a biological system in which three entities—human, parasite, and mosquito—have been co-evolving for centuries. Generally, the stated goal of international efforts to combat malaria has moved from eradication to minimizing its impact, even though the idea that eradication may be within reach has started to gain currency again (Bill and Melinda Gates Foundation 2007). Concomitantly, propositions on how to address malaria changed from approaches that rely on single biomedical tools to those that rely on a combination of measures, and engage a variety of different actors.

As the following section will show, the evolution of international approaches to malaria control can be divided into three phases and shows important similarities to the evolution of responses to tuberculosis described in the previous section. Thus, first approaches to malaria control were vertical in structure and relied on newly discovered scientific tools and knowledge that were thought to be effective in controlling or even eradicating it. After these efforts had failed, a phase followed during which attention to malaria decreased, until it was perceived as resurging and represented as being transnational in nature. A period followed during which horizontal approaches, delivered through the state with support of the WHO, were thought to be the right solution to the problem. And, finally, much as in the case of tuberculosis, the international health community ended up concluding that malaria could not be effectively addressed by a Westphalian arrangement of national and international institutions, leading the way to partnerships being advocated as the superior type of governance for malaria control. The following section will trace in detail these changes in scientific and public health thinking that happened through time.

1920s–1960s: Silver Bullets

Malaria came onto the agenda of international health cooperation in the early 1920s. At the time, it was still prevalent in some European countries, including Italy, Greece, and the Balkans. The 1920s–1940s were marked by a public health controversy over the right method to address the disease between the League of Nation's Malaria Commission and the mighty Rockefeller Foundation, which Stapleton has described in detail.[15] He points out that with its far-reaching global activities,[16] the Rockefeller Foundation was not just a key driver of scientific developments at the time, but was at the core of a "revolution in malaria control" happening at the time.

Essentially, the League of Nation's Malaria Commission held that the best way to control malaria was the combination of quinine with the spraying of pyrethrum in houses, combined with social measures to improve living conditions (Bruce-Chwatt and de Zulueta 1980, 169). In contrast, the International Health Board (IHB) and later the Rockefeller Foundation itself pioneered a new approach that was exclusively based on the killing of mosquito larvae with a chemical named "Paris Green" (Stapleton 2004).[17] These malaria programs required in-depth study of the local conditions of the vector—regarded as "scientific, experimental and temporary," they aimed at vector eradication (Stapleton 2004). Thus, the Rockefeller approach promised a silver bullet to end an ancient scourge.

The controversy, which can be interpreted as a competition between a vertical approach with the aim to eradicate and a horizontal approach with the aim to control, was later won by the vertical fraction. In the course of the 1930s and 1940s, the Rockefeller Foundation came to be seen as one of the major contributors to successful malaria control all over the world, and especially in Europe (Bruce-Chwatt and de Zulueta 1980, 171).[18] The foundation's approach, with its focus on technical tools and its belief that temporary, scientific intervention can solve the problem, is thought to have helped pave the way for the later focus on eradication by the WHO (Stapleton 2004). However, according to Bruce-Chwatt and de Zulueta, it became clear by the mid-1940s that this approach, which was based on decreasing or eliminating mosquitoes, could not realistically be applied in vast malarious regions of many developing countries (Bruce-Chwatt and de Zulueta 1980, 172).

It was the discovery, in 1948, of the inexpensive, synthetic insecticide *dichlorodiphenyltrichloroethane* (DDT) that changed the pendulum toward eradication. Evidence from Greece and Sardinia[19] indicating that DDT was effective for malaria control if sprayed indoors for a limited time period led the WHO to announce a Global Malaria Eradication Campaign at the eighth World Health Assembly in 1955 (Bruce-Chwatt and de Zulueta 1980). As Trigg and Kondrachine point out, eradication, as a concept, "hinged on the idea that the transmission of malaria in a community would be interrupted if a sufficient number of adult mosquitoes were killed before the parasite development in the vector was completed"; this thinking was based on mathematical projections that suggested that the biological cycle of *plasmodium* could be fully discontinued with the help of DDT and larvicides (Trigg and Kondrachine 1998). It seems thus fair to say that it was, in its structure and design, a "vertical" program, which relied on the idea that biomedicine was transportable across national boundaries and applicable regardless of geographic and cultural context. The very word "campaign" suggests a time-limited effort.

Its title also suggested global reach, but in fact, that was misleading. The global eradication machinery was never deployed in most of sub-Saharan Africa, with few exceptions[20]—malaria experts believed that in those regions, levels of malaria transmission were too high and health infrastructure too feeble to make sufficient headway against the disease (Trigg and Kondrachine 1998).

By the end of the 1960s, malaria had been successfully eradicated in developed countries.[21] However, reexamining the results of the overall effort, the

22nd World Health Assembly in Boston came to the conclusion that the goal of eradicating malaria was not attainable, mainly due to weak public infrastructure in many regions (Trigg and Kondrachine 1998). The assembly officially changed the focus of global malaria efforts to controlling its transmission (Bruce-Chwatt and de Zulueta 1980).

1970s–1980s: Malaria "Resurgence"

In a pattern that reminds us of the tuberculosis case, the perceived failure of the eradication campaign first led to an apparent loss of interest on the part of the international health community. Funding for antimalarial programs dropped substantially, and the WHO drastically reduced its technical staff in affected countries, prompting the ironic comment "Since they couldn't eradicate malaria, they eradicated the [malaria researchers]" (Balter 2000). The economic crisis in the early 1970s led to increases in the price of insecticides, antimalarial drugs, and shipping costs, which further hampered malaria programs in many developing countries (Trigg and Kondrachine 1998).

After the end of the eradication campaign, malaria resurged in those regions of Asia and South America where transmission had been successfully reduced (Nchinda 1998). In Africa, where eradication had never been attempted, rates rose throughout the 1970 and 1980s, due to a number of factors, including population movements, climatic changes, and resistance to antimalarials and insecticides (Nchinda 1998). Chloroquine-resistant *falciparum* malaria had spread throughout the world (Wernsdorfer 1991). Malaria came to be regarded as intimately linked with globalization. At the beginning of the 1990s, it was estimated that there were 300–500 million cases of malaria each year and that 1.5–2.7 million people died from it, with 90 percent of its burden confined to sub-Saharan Africa (Rugemalila, Wanga, and Wen 2006).

1990s: Control Through the Primary Health Care Approach

In the second half of the 1990s, malaria slowly regained its status as an international priority. As the following paragraphs will show, the changed representation of malaria combined with the perceived failure of the eradication campaign produced a paradigm change—international cooperation on malaria, it was argued, cannot expect to conquer malaria with single technological fixes, but must combine a variety of tools, pay attention to local ecological and socioeconomic conditions, and aim for control rather than eradication.

In 1992, a WHO-proposed Ministerial Conference on Malaria held in Amsterdam adopted World Declaration on Malaria with a Global Malaria Control Strategy (World Health Organization 1992). Efforts were made to anchor the new strategy at all levels of existing national, regional, and UN governance. Thus, both the Declaration and the Strategy were later endorsed by World Health Assembly in 1993, by the United Nations General Assembly in 1994, and by the Organization of African Unity in 1997 (Trigg and Kondrachine 1998). In their analysis of malaria control in the 1990s, Trigg and Kondrachine made the argument that it differed substantially from previous approaches in that it was a "change of emphasis from highly prescriptive, centralized control programmes to flexible, cost-effective and sustainable programmes adapted to local conditions and responding to local needs" (Trigg and Kondrachine 1998). Among the different components of the strategy (World Health Organization 1992), three stand out: first, the new strategy was going to be implemented through primary health care systems; second, international and local research, both basic and applied, would be central to its success—therefore, local research capabilities needed to be strengthened and international research networks enhanced; third, malaria control would have to be integrated with work in other sectors, such as education and environment, and that it needed to actively engage communities in the control efforts.

The idea that governments in the developing countries needed to lead both malaria research and malaria control found additional institutional expression in the second half of the 1990s. In 1995, the U.S. National Institutes of Health Malaria convened major research institutions, including France's Institut Pasteur and the British Wellcome Trust and Medical Research Council, to devise a strategy for invigorating and strengthening cooperation on malaria research globally (Mons et al. 1998). This effort led to the founding, in 1997, of the Multilateral Initiative on Malaria (MIM), by a group of over 150 European and African scientists and representatives of the world's major funders of malaria research (Bruno et al. 1997; Mons et al. 1998). The initiative was to build on existing global research programs, including, for example, WHO's Special Programme for Research and Training in Tropical Diseases (TDR), to build "networks of excellence" that would be "unrestricted by geography" (Mons et al. 1998); through it, African malaria scientists were going to gain access to means and capabilities for malaria research and collaboration with the North (and vice versa), because "continuing dominance by Northern partners does not yield lasting partnerships" (Mons et al. 1998). Thus, knowledge generation about malaria was considered crucial to efforts at controlling the disease; it is also seen as freely traveling across national boundaries.

Overall, we can discern in these developments a shift from a top-down, centralized way of controlling malaria to one that gives weight to local action, and an increasing emphasis to invigorate and integrate local knowledge production. Science and scientific activity are at the core of global malaria policy. However, the overall approach to malaria control at that time was still clearly "Westphalian" in the sense that national governments, with support from the WHO and other UN agencies and from the international scientific establishment, are conceptualized as the main actors through which malaria control is delivered.

Roll Back Malaria: The Era of Partnerships

In July 1998, Gro Harlem Brundtland took office as the new Director-General of the WHO. Brundtland is credited for moving malaria back to the very top of the global health agenda (Balter 2000; "Reversing the failures of Roll Back Malaria" 2005). In May 1998, she announced a new initiative called "Roll Back Malaria" (RBM). Its goal was to reduce malaria-related mortality worldwide by 50 percent over the coming decade, and then by another 50 percent by the year 2015 (Nabarro and Tayler 1998). In line with the changed representation of malaria as a transnational issue, RBM was conceptualized as a global effort that would integrate in its strategy and workings the adaptation to major emerging transnational trends. For example, it would take into account climate change, human migration, and the emergence of resistance to commonly used antimalarial tools (Nabarro and Tayler 1998).

The public image of malaria was now one of a disease intimately intertwined with globalization. In 1999, the BBC printed an article that cited the WHO warning that, as a consequence of global warming, the disease was on its way back to Great Britain and Europe ("Global warming disease warning" 1999). The conception of malaria as a force affecting society and impacting economic development and social life had become more and more nuanced with the economics profession having turned its eye to it in the context of international development (see, for example, Sachs 1997, 2001; Sachs and Malaney 2002). The representation of malaria as a disease affecting every aspect of social life in Africa, from child and maternal mortality to adult well-being and labor productivity, is illustrated in the following quote from a 2000 editorial in the *Bulletin of the WHO*:

Malaria kills a child somewhere in the world every 30 seconds. The majority of the deaths it causes occur in Africa. Malaria is a major factor in Africa's high rate of infant and maternal mortality, of low birth weight, of school absenteeism, and of low productivity in farming and other work. It afflicts primarily the poor, who tend to live in malaria-endemic areas and in dwellings that offer little or no protection against mosquitoes. By sapping people's health, strength and productivity, malaria further marginalizes and impoverishes them.

(Alnwick 2000)

Like "Stop TB," RBM was constructed as a horizontal program (Breman 2000), designed to strengthen national action ("Round Table Discussion: Rolling back malaria: action or rhetoric?" 2000). Like "Stop TB," it was made up of over 90 entities. And like Stop TB, some of its proponents saw it as the start of a "societal movement" with the aim to put a halt to the disease ("Round Table Discussion: Rolling back malaria: action or rhetoric?" 2000). Commentaries from the time of its inception suggest that it was set up to counteract all of the perceived mistakes of the past. An article in *Science Magazine* explained in great detail the differences to previous WHO efforts. For example, it would not be a separate entity, but would work from within national health systems; it would combine social and biomedical research to generate new antimalarial tools, and not make the mistake to over-depend on any single malaria control instrument; maybe most importantly, it would not be a one-time effort, but a sustained activity, global in reach, yet adapted to regional necessities (Nabarro and Tayler 1998). Thus, as in the case of tuberculosis, the new partnership was presented as an institutional solution that could address both the "transnational" and the "local" qualities of malaria.

Initial reactions to RBM were mixed. Optimists stressed that malaria was a preventable and curable disease, and argued that, therefore, RBM could make a dent in it (Nabarro and Mendis 2000). Optimists expected the program to revolutionize malaria control and set an example for other complicated health issues, such as TB control and health problems during motherhood, and to set "new standards for partnership between the public and private sectors" in the health domain (Nabarro and Tayler 1998). More skeptical voices pointed to past failures and cautioned against high expectations (Druilhe 2000; Greenwood 2000; Kilama 2000). There were also reservations about whether or not the tools necessary to make a dent in malaria were really available, whether a horizontal partnership could strengthen malaria control, whether it was possible to adequately assess its performance, and whether or not the necessary funding would be made available (see, for example, "Round Table Discussion: Rolling back malaria: action or rhetoric?" 2000). But overall, leading experts argued that notwithstanding the perceived past failures, the WHO was the agency that combined the needed "moral authority" with the necessary "technical know-how" to lead the global fight against malaria (Balter 2000). RBM was later credited for raising awareness and political support for malaria and as having caused a substantial increase in international spending ("Reversing the failures of Roll Back Malaria" 2005).

As was the case for tuberculosis, international approaches to malaria control thus evolved over time from centralized, government-driven programs (vertical and horizontal) with technical support from the WHO to a much more loose notion of a global partnership between state and nonstate actors.

HIV/AIDS: The New Pandemic

This section focuses on the evolution of responses to HIV/AIDS before the inception of the Global Fund. In contrast to tuberculosis and malaria, which had been well known for centuries, HIV/AIDS was a new disease that shocked and puzzled the Western world by appearing, out of nowhere it seemed, at the end of the second millennium. It first needed to be described, named, and understood. In the Western world, the initial image of HIV/AIDS as a disease of homosexuals, hemophiliacs, and heroin users changed to that of a condition that affected discrete, small subpopulation of promiscuous individuals only, and was therefore not going to threaten the stability of industrialized countries. The fact that developing countries, and especially societies in sub-Saharan Africa, were experiencing an entirely different situation became evident in the mid-1990s, mainly through the work of the international public health establishment.

With the changing representation of HIV/AIDS, approaches to addressing it also changed. As in the cases of tuberculosis and malaria, there was a shift from WHO-run organizational structure to a notion of cross-sectoral partnership. However, in 1996, WHO's Global Programme on Aids was replaced not with an equivalent WHO-led partnership like "Stop TB" or "Roll Back Malaria," but with its own, separate UN agency. HIV/AIDS had attained global status on the basis of its rapid spread and the severity with which it affected developing country populations. However, in the absence of an affordable therapy for the disease, the aid community emphasized approaches to halting its spread through multisectoral collaboration. Barton Gellman has written in *The Washington Post* an excellent account of the emergence of HIV/AIDS and the evolution in contemporary thinking about HIV/AIDS at the WHO and in the aid community (Gellman 2000a, 2000b, 2000c, 2000d). This section as well as the next chapter relies on his account on multiple occasions.

Beginnings: WHO's Global Program on HIV/AIDS

The first WHO meeting to assess the global AIDS situation was held in November 1983, and marked the start of global AIDS surveillance (World Health Organization 1983a, 1983b, 1983c). Two years after the first cases had appeared in different spots across the globe, the supranational public health establishment was turning an observing eye on the new disease. About 3,000 cases of AIDS (defined by the U.S. Centers for Disease Control as a set of the disease's hallmark clinical symptoms) had been detected mostly in the United States and Western Europe, although—as the first December issue of the WHO's *Weekly Epidemiological Record* noted—"cases [of AIDS] are now appearing in a number of developing countries and else-where" (World Health Organization 1983a, 369). The origins of the disease were still unknown—its viral origins were to be discovered only a year later— and, needless to say, a treatment was not available. Thus, HIV/AIDS initially received attention at the supranational level not on the basis of available biomedical tools or pervasive presence in developing countries, but because of its unknown origins, rapid spread, and fatal outcome—it was perceived as a potential threat that needed to be monitored.

And indeed, the institutionalization of continuous surveillance at WHO-level did not mean that HIV/AIDS was automatically considered a global health priority. Global HIV infection rates were still overall low. Many regarded the disease mainly as a threat to homosexuals, drug users, and sub-populations of promiscuous individuals. Furthermore, an effective prevention or therapy was unavailable. Halfdan Mahler, then Director-General of the WHO, held that other diseases, like tuberculosis and malaria, were much more pressing (Gellman 2000b).

Early hints that the disease was rapidly spreading through heterosexual pathways in Africa existed, but were initially dismissed. Gellman describes the efforts of a group of Western researchers to investigate an apparently het-erosexual spread of the new disease in what was then Zaire (see Gellman 2000b). The team was led by the Belgian physician Peter Piot, one of the co-discoverers of the Ebola virus in 1976 and later the first head of UNAIDS. Gellman's account shows that they had been alerted by a local medical practitioner—Bila Kapita, who headed the internal medicine department at Mama Yemo hospital in Kinshasa, was concerned about an increasing num-ber of young men and women dying from a devastating immune deficiency that was locally referred to as "slim disease"; he had read reports of a new fatal immune disease observed in California in the scientific literature and wanted to know whether he was seeing cases of it among his patients. According to Gellman, Piot was shocked by the epidemiological pattern he was see-ing: "There were so many women, it said to me it's heterosexual . . . That means everybody's at risk . . . Until then I never thought a whole country, a whole population, could be involved" (Gellman 2000b). It is interesting to note that the initiative for this investigation came from a local medi-cal expert, who was accessing knowledge in the global scientific literature. The institutions of the international scientific establishment, including the publication of peer-reviewed studies, functioned as a pathway through which the local and the global could be connected and could become the target of international scientific work and collaboration.

However, the same pathways were not working when Piot and his colleagues wanted to transport to the global level the threatening scenario they were seeing in Kinshasa. As Gellman (2000b) further describes, Piot and his colleagues had immense difficulties in convincing their peers that HIV/AIDS was a heterosexual disease—a paper they had written on the basis of about 40 male and female cases they had seen in Kinshasa was rejected by a series of scientific journals; the reviewers insisted the authors had "overlooked an alternate path of transmission." And even at the first international AIDS conference in Atlanta held in 1985, Gellman writes that there were mainly negative reactions to the work: "people . . . said this is nonsense," he quotes Piot. Piot et al.'s evidence, made on the basis of a relatively small number of closely observed cases, was apparently not sufficient proof to convince international experts of something the world absolutely did not want to believe: that HIV can rapidly spread through heterosexual sex. More evidence, quantitative and qualitative, would be needed until their hypothesis could become part of the global body of knowledge about HIV/AIDS that later became the basis for public health action.

This changed only slowly, with the continued efforts of international public health experts to make visible the African epidemic to the eye of the supranational health institution in Geneva. According to Gellman, this was achieved when, in 1986, the WHO's chief of infectious diseases, Fakhry Assaad, brought a young physician named Jonathan Mann to Geneva, who had been leading follow-up work to Piot's studies through Projet SIDA, a joint U.S., Belgian, and Zairian project, and who was convinced that AIDS was of "transcendental importance" (Gellman 2000b). Mann was to head WHO's first AIDS program and was arguably one of the most dedicated and influential thinkers and activists in the history of the disease. Gellman describes how, as early as 1986, Mann connected HIV's rapid spread in Kinshasa with certain social conditions—poverty, oppression, urban migration, and violence—and was convinced that HIV/AIDS was unamenable to the prevalent biomedical disease control paradigm; he saw discrimination as a primary cause of the epidemic and was convinced that HIV/AIDS would spread rapidly; at a news conference at the United Nations headquarters in November 1986, he declared: "We stand nakedly in front of a pandemic as mortal as any pandemic there has ever been" (Gellman 2000b). By proposing that discrimination was a cause (not just an effect) of HIV/AIDS, Mann was proposing a representation of HIV/AIDS that was not purely biomedical in nature.

Mann was heard by Mahler and others at the WHO and the subsequent years, 1986–1987, brought a significant increase in political attention and funding for AIDS. Mahler instituted a new Global Program on AIDS (GPA), which reported directly to him, thereby ignoring the hierarchical structures of which other WHO programs were expected to be part of it and putting Mann in the lead (Gellman 2000b), a signal that the disease was moving up on the list of the health agency's priorities. A session of the UN General Assembly was devoted to AIDS in 1987. At that meeting, AIDS was not only declared to be "global," but was also presented as a problem that had important economic, social, cultural, and political dimensions (Mann 1987b).

Under Mann's and Mahler's leadership, the GPA retained political momentum for a while. Based on its structure as the program of a UN agency, a key role it took was to mobilize national health agencies in its member states. In January 1988, the GPA convened 118 health ministers in London to discuss a common strategy toward AIDS, which led to the London Declaration on AIDS Prevention emphasizing education and human rights as key factors to preventing an epidemic (Hadlington 1988). In May 1987, the 40th World Health Assembly approved the new program's first *Global Strategy on AIDS* (Mann 1987a). By November of that year, more than 62,000 cases of AIDS were reported to the WHO from 127 countries (Mann 1987b). In the absence of a treatment, the program's focus was on the prevention of HIV, and its aim was to support national responses to AIDS and to coordinate the international response. In 1988, World AIDS Day was introduced (Goldsmith 1988; "World AIDS Day" 1988).

International scientific cooperation on HIV/AIDS also intensified. In April 1985, the first International Conference on AIDS was held in Atlanta, attended by over 3,000 people from over 50 nations (World Health Organization 1985). The language of the memorandum that WHO published on the basis of the meeting is instructive. It reports about 11,000 cases of HIV, predominantly in the industrialized world (of which more than 80 percent were in the United States), and notes that "recent information indicates that AIDS may be a serious public health problem in tropical Africa," with "estimated incidence rates in some central African cities . . . comparable to those in New York or San Francisco" (World Health Organization 1985). The idea that HIV/AIDS could spread heterosexually in a major way was not widely accepted. A quote from *The New York Times* in the same year also reflects a cautious assessment of the validity of that idea:

> Some experts are skeptical that AIDS will spread as rapidly among heterosexuals as it has among homosexuals. Yet other experts, taking their cues from data

emerging from preliminary studies from Africa showing equal sex distribution among males and females, are less sure.

(Altman 1985)

In September 1986, a therapy for HIV/AIDS appeared on the horizon with the discovery that *azidothymidine* (AZT) could decelerate the progression of AIDS (Yarchoan et al. 1986). This implied that science was starting to yield tools to control the disease. But even before the discovery of AZT, based on epidemiological observations, the view had been transported in the press that the patterns of the spread of HIV differed substantially between certain African nations and the Western world, with a large-scale heterosexual spread of HIV/AIDS unlikely in the United States and Europe (see, for example, Wade 1988; Gellman 2000b).

Mann and others had categorized the geographic spread in three patterns (Von Reyn and Mann 1987), which supported this view: pattern I was observed mainly in the United States and Europe, and was primarily characterized by homosexual and bisexual intercourse, injection drug use, and, to a small extent, contaminated blood supplies. Consequently, it showed low infection rates among women, and therefore low mother-to-child transmission rates. Pattern II was prevalent in Africa and Haiti, and was mainly based on heterosexual transmission. In this pattern, the seroprevalence was overall elevated compared to in pattern I, the infection rates in men and women were equal, and there were substantial amounts of mother-to-child transmission. Pattern III, prevalent in Asia and the Middle East, was mainly based on injection drug use and prostitution. This classification of the epidemiological patterns of HIV/AIDS was a way of creating order in the disorder that the new disease had given rise to.

It is worth noting that this 1987 publication is already very close to the way that HIV/AIDS was later represented and described in these regions. However, to many of those shaping public health at the time, the evidence was too scant to convince them that Mann et al.'s "pattern II" was the correct representation of HIV/AIDS in Africa and should therefore form the basis of international policy in that region. Thus, some internal experts at WHO had started arguing that the size and importance of the GPA were out of proportion compared to the few actually proven cases of AIDS at the time (Hilts 1990; Gellman 2000b).

In the second half of the 1980s, the pendulum swung in the direction of the skeptics, and as a result, support for the GPA decreased. A leadership change at WHO withdrew from Mann the support he had previously had from the top of the organization. Hiroshi Nakajima was elected Director-General in 1998. When asked about HIV/AIDS, he famously said: "ah, don't talk to me about AIDS. I have malaria, a much bigger killer of people, on my hands" (Gellman 2000b). Their cooperation lasted only two years and, according to contemporary accounts, ended in an outright clash: in 1990, Mann resigned from GPA after openly accusing Nakajima of obstructing his efforts in an interview with the French newspaper *Le Monde* (Hilts 1990; Gellman 2000b). Nakajima appointed Michael Merson, formerly director of the WHO program for diarrheal diseases control, as successor ("U.N. body appoints new AIDS director" 1990).

The Creation of UNAIDS

In the late 1980s, HIV/AIDS coverage in the press became more and more dramatic. For example, in 1988, an article in *The New York Times* reported that 5 percent of Congo's population was infected with HIV, painting grim scenarios for the countries it labeled "Africa's AIDS belt"—Zaire, Zambia, and Tancan Republic (Brooke 1988). By the beginning of the 1990s, there were news reports of infection rates among adults of up to 20 percent from some large African cities (Eckholm and Tierney 1990). But key donors and decision makers in the international community were not convinced that a pandemic was about to decimate African populations. In 1991, an Interagency Intelligence Memorandum with the stark title "The Global AIDS Disaster" was distributed among classified channels in the U.S. administration; its authors foresaw 45 million HIV infections by 2000, mostly in the south of Africa, but did not receive any serious attention (Gellman 2000b). When a British scientist named Roy Anderson at the Imperial College in London predicted, in 1992, that because of AIDS, certain African populations would start declining within two decades, this was contrary to projections of major agencies and donors of the time, who foresaw a slowdown, but no decline, in population growth (Perlez 1992). In 1992, World Bank review of its agenda on AIDS and other sexually transmitted infections declared that while AIDS was a serious threat to health, it "should not dominate the Bank's health agenda in Africa" (World Bank 2005).

With time, the representation of HIV/AIDS as a force affecting the societal fabric of African nations became more nuanced and explicit. A 1993 WHO study was reported in the press showing that 60 percent of new infections in Africa were happening in individuals under age 25 ("U.N. Agency Reports AIDS Virus Spreading Very Quickly in Africa" 1993). News stories focused increasingly on the effects of HIV/AIDS on young people (Altman 2000), teachers, doctors, and engineers (Eckholm and Tierney 1990) as victims of HIV/AIDS. In their vignettes from African cities, journalists described a situation where fear reigned and where recent deaths and funerals were the main topic of conversations at meetings among people (see, for example, Eckholm 1990). As the head of the WHO's regional office for Africa, Ebrahim Samba put it to the Associated Press: "You go to parts of Uganda now and see orphaned children and elderly people, and in between there's nothing. It doesn't take a genius to see that's a disaster for the economy and for society" (Nullis 1995). Increasingly, the representation of HIV/AIDS thus shifted from one that listed its statistics at the population level toward one that mobilized existing evidence to emphasize social, economic, and behavioral effects at the subnational and individual levels.

The WHO also made the argument for action. At the 1993 AIDS conference in Berlin, Mann's successor Michael Merson presented a first cost estimate for global AIDS prevention: US$ 2.5 billion, or an equivalent of about 20 times global spending on HIV/AIDS, would be needed in total to prevent half of the 20 million new cases expected by the year 2000, he said, quoting to Gellman, and added: "the world can find this kind of money when it wants to" (Gellman 2000b). But with the argument that "health" was too narrow an angle for addressing such a broad, multifactorial problem, also came a perception that the institutional structure of the GPA was not apt to addressing HIV/AIDS. Public health officials and donor governments started to push for a joint UN program on AIDS to be instituted in its place. According to accounts from the period, the establishment of UNAIDS only came about after heated struggle between the UN agencies, during which Michael Merson's program was accused of being too focused on the biomedical dimensions of AIDS and inadequately capable of engaging at the grassroots levels in affected countries (Nullis 1995). Administrative battles over responsibility and funding lasted two years before the program was officially launched in January 1996 (Gellman 2000b).

Thus, by the mid-1990s, HIV/AIDS had come to be seen as a heterosexual epidemic with the potential to endanger the fabric of certain societies, especially in sub-Saharan Africa. But in contrast to tuberculosis and malaria, for which large, WHO-led multilateral partnerships were later instituted, HIV/AIDS received its own UN agency to lead and coordinate a multisectoral approach that could draw on other UN agencies—for example, the WHO; the UN Children's Fund; the UN Population Fund; the UN Educational, Scientific, and Cultural Organization (UNESCO); the UN Development Program (UNDP); and the World Bank. Great emphasis was laid on the importance of involving local communities and NGOs in the response to the disease. UNAIDS was conceptualized as a "thin layer at the top which can take innovative steps to reach the grassroots" (Awuonda 1995). It was hoped that the integration of the HIV/AIDS-related components of these agencies would enable the United Nations to address some of the perceived gaps between the grassroots and government levels, for example, on preventive measures such as condom distribution and education (Nullis 1995).

However, while the creation of a separate UN agency for HIV/AIDS can certainly be interpreted as an elevation in the importance of the disease on the international agenda, UNAIDS hardly represented an overall progress in terms of funding. Its proposed biennial budget was US$ 120–140 million for 1996–1997 (McGregor 1995), which represented no increase compared to the US$ 130 the WHO had spent (Gellman 2000b). Moreover, the program's co-sponsors dramatically decreased the resources they spent on AIDS: the United Nations Children's Fund (UNICEF) lowered its investments from US$ 45 million to US$ 10 million, and World Bank loans for HIV/AIDS-related programs decreased from US$ 50 million to US$ 10 million (Gellman 2000b).

Most importantly, there were no plans to make HIV testing or treatment widely available in developing countries. According to Gellman, many development organizations attempted to shield their resources from the growing AIDS epidemic throughout much of the 1990s (Gellman 2000b).[22] Behind this reluctance, he asserts, was the idea that since HIV testing could not be followed up with an effective treatment, it would only create demand for other services that neither local governments nor outside agencies could pay for. Thus, he reports that Duff Gillespie, who was overseeing AIDS assistance at the United States Agency for International Development at the time, explained in a memorandum the lack of political will to fight AIDS in the donor community at the time with three major factors: the epidemic's "important disadvantages," including the lack of tools that "directly and invariably" prevented transmission; the absence of a cure; and the lack of "an inherently sympathetic victim" (Gellman 2000b).

Conclusion

In this chapter I have traced the institutionalization of responses to tuberculosis, malaria, and HIV/AIDS at the supranational level in order to understand how they came to be regarded as global. The chapter shows that a number of different factors can play a role in determining global status. These include the distribution and impact of a disease, the speed of its spread, the severity of its outcome, and the availability of tools to prevent and/or cure it. When combinations of these factors were present, "globalization" occurred on the basis of biomedicine, on the basis of a postulated universal human right to health, or on the basis of transnational spread (and, by extension, threat) of a given disease. The biomedical framework provides a relatively straightforward identity to the patient as a global citizen in a treatment regime, on the basis that biology is independent of nationality. However, as the example of HIV/AIDS shows, the same process appears more difficult when no clear cause and/or no defined intervention is available.

Tuberculosis and malaria are archetypical examples of twentieth-century public health cooperation. When antibiotics and vaccines appeared, they were part of a range of infectious diseases that were now regarded as preventable and curable and were initially targeted in top-down vertical disease control programs at the WHO. Over time, the representation of these two diseases changed fundamentally as they became seen as not just biomedical issues but also complex biomedical, social, economic, and cultural issues. Tuberculosis came to be regarded as a matter of the successful organizational management of large-scale programs ("scale-up"). Malaria came to be seen as a biological system in which humans, parasites, and mosquitoes co-evolve. In both cases, the WHO's efforts to eliminate and/or control the diseases were seen as hampered by an inability to account for local diversity and to connect to the grassroots levels.

In contrast to tuberculosis and malaria, HIV/AIDS initially achieved global status, in the absence of prevention or cure, purely on the basis of its sudden emergence, rapid spread, and fatal outcome. A vertical program was instituted at the WHO for the purpose of surveillance. HIV/AIDS moved up on the list of global health priorities when its rapid heterosexual spread in some regions of sub-Saharan Africa gave rise to the argument that it was a threat to the stability of entire nation-states. In 1996, UNAIDS was created, reflecting the belief that HIV/AIDS was not adequately addressed as a *biomedical* issue, nor as a multifactorial *health* issue to be addressed under the aegis of the WHO, but rather represented a cross-cutting development problem requiring a coordinated response from all departments of the United Nations. As a consequence, HIV/AIDS received its own UN agency.

Over the course of the 1980s and 1990s, all three diseases came to be regarded as transnational and as intimately intertwined with globalization. With this new representation, the dominant paradigm of international health cooperation shifted away from a division of responsibilities along the lines of national governments toward the idea that partnerships between governments, intergovernmental organizations, and a variety of nonstate actors would yield superior solutions to these long-standing global health issues. The partnership is presented not only as a response to the challenges posed by the "transnationality" but also as a solution to the need to respond to local diversity. This is evidenced in the fact that "Stop TB" and "Roll Back Malaria" were conceptualized as "social movements." The underlying assumption is that the state is not always able to reach down to the grassroots level (that is, the local communities and civil society organizations) of its own sovereign domain. The patient is transformed from a *subject* of health policy to whom interventions are delivered through top-down national programs to an *agent* that actively takes part in health improvement inside a system that is connected across local, regional, and global levels. This represents a challenge to the Westphalian principle of noninterference, which assumes the sovereignty of national governments in all matters concerning their citizens.

By the end of the 1990s, both malaria and tuberculosis were instituted in the form of partnerships, Stop TB and Roll Back Malaria. Their stated goal was to make treatment available to patients in all afflicted countries. HIV/AIDS had been given its own UN agency, but this elevation in terms of importance on the international agenda was not matched with a declared intent to treat patients in need with AZT, which was available at the time. The therapy's high price and lack of curative effect prevented global health actors from promising antiretroviral therapy to all HIV/AIDS patients in the same way. Evidently, when a treatment is considered too expensive, the biomedical framework doesn't suffice to confer global status, even when the severity and distribution of a disease are not under question. As the next chapter will show, fundamental changes in the scientific, political, and economic spheres were necessary to change that.

CHAPTER 3

The Global Fund Experiment

In March 2002, the Global Fund to Fight Aids, Tuberculosis and Malaria announced its first round of funding—close to US$ 2 billion to support developing countries in their efforts to prevent and treat HIV/AIDS (Ramsay 2002). This was an important moment in the history of global health. At the turn of the millennium, the large-scale distribution of antiretrovirals (ARVs) to patients in poor countries had still been considered prohibitively expensive, technically unfeasible, and generally impossible. No actor in the health domain wanted to take the responsibility for funding such an endeavor. Only two years later, the prices of ARVs had fallen by a factor of 25; international funding for the prevention and treatment of HIV/AIDS had increased from millions to several billions of U.S. dollars, and the international community had set up a new financing mechanism outside of the United Nations system to channel these resources directly to developing countries. Thus, an unprecedented increase in resources for a single health issue was combined with a fundamental shift in the global health institutional landscape, away from a system in which the multilateral institutions provided mainly technical advice and advocacy on HIV/AIDS to one in which new models of collective action, including public-private partnerships, are taking an active role in priority setting and funding of prevention and treatment.

The Global Fund promotes the basic idea that *all* HIV/AIDS patients should have access to the same standard of antiretroviral therapy, regardless of which nation they happen to live in.[1] This chapter is devoted to two main questions. First, why do we have a Global Fund—how did this new actor emerge in the global health domain? Second, what does the appearance of this large new body mean for the interaction between existing players in the global health domain?

In order to answer these questions, I trace in this chapter the emergence of the Global Fund between 2000 and 2002. It shows that the Global Fund is the result of intense political struggles over the responsibility for the provision of antiretroviral therapy to HIV/AIDS patients in developing countries. These struggles were triggered at the end of the 1990s, when important changes in the scientific and political domains generated a unique constellation of local and global actors that would change the way the world thought about HIV/AIDS. While the clashes between civil society and the pharmaceutical industry over the prices of antiretroviral medicines were arguably the most visible aspect of these political conflicts, the chapter will show that they actually took place simultaneously on many different local and global stages, involving not just the pharmaceutical industry and civil society but also national governments, the international scientific community, and multilateral organizations.

In the course of these struggles, the *representation* of HIV/AIDS changed fundamentally. HIV/AIDS had always been regarded as a serious public health issue at the national level, but now it was reinterpreted as a threat to global security that required not only immediate action but also new forms of institutions. This "globalization" of HIV/AIDS happened through three interdependent pathways. The first is *science*. Biomedical and social scientists in academia and other organizations were linked cross-nationally through activities that ranged from the generation of scientific knowledge about HIV/AIDS and the conduction of international clinical trials to advocacy with national governments. The second globalizing pathway is the *market*. National and multinational pharmaceutical companies were expanding their activities across national boundaries, functioning as powerful standard-setting forces as they worked to protect their domestic markets while extending their revenue-generating domains into the developing world. The third globalizing factor is the growing *transnational civil society movement* that had allied across boundaries, demanding access to antiretroviral treatment for patients in developing countries since the late 1990s, arguing that health is a human right that knows no borders.

The issue of *mother-to-child transmission* of HIV served as connecting thread among these multiple sites of contestation. Simultaneously local and global, particular and abstract, the threat that HIV posed to the unborn/newborn child played a central role in the ongoing political struggles. Over time, the child figured as the epitome of the "innocent victim," whose blamelessness was undisputed across national boundaries and whose protection no one could seriously object to, and also as the "future marauding orphan," who was bound to become the agent of a transnational security nightmare and eventually whose slide into poverty, desperation, and possible violence needed to be prevented at all cost.

These different yet intertwined forces combined in multiple ways to move the plight of poor HIV/AIDS patients to the global level. A first formal turning point happened in 2000, when the UN Security Council declared HIV/AIDS a human security issue. A second formal turning point happened in 2001, when the UN General Assembly declared that all HIV/AIDS patients, regardless of their nationality, should have access to ARVs as a matter of global priority. In this process of reinterpretation, existing national and international norms in domains as different as politics, trade, intellectual property, clinical medicine, and ethics also had to be negotiated and renegotiated. The result was a fundamental reordering of the way the world addressed the HIV/AIDS epidemic and a fundamental redefinition of responsibilities among local and global players in the health domain: for the first time, local actors were able to directly access a financing mechanism outside of the United Nations for grants (not loans) in direct support of their HIV/AIDS programs.

Biopolitical Constellations: Profits of the Rich Versus Plight of the Poor

As the previous chapter has shown, the provision of antiretroviral therapy to HIV/AIDS patients in developing countries was not part of the international development agenda in the mid- and late 1990s. This was not because there was much doubt left about the seriousness of the HIV/AIDS epidemic in Africa. The epidemic had been rapidly spreading in developing countries, especially sub-Saharan Africa, for more than 15 years. In 1996, 21 million adults were reported to be living with the virus, and 7,500 new infections were thought to happen every day (Simons 1996). Based on assessments by the UN and other experts, who were predicting that HIV/AIDS would severely impact the population growth of African countries, its terrible impact in that region was no longer questioned, but firmly asserted in news coverage of the time (see, for example, "Severe AIDS effects seen on population of Africa" 1996; Ibrahim 1998). But humanity seemed poorly equipped to deal with this terrible scourge. AZT and other single drug regimens, then the mainstay of antiretroviral therapy, slowed down the virus, but not substantially enough to be considered a dramatic breakthrough for HIV/AIDS patients (several months to a few years) (Elhaggar 1993). They were also prohibitively expensive at more than US$ 10,000 or more per patient per year (Gellman 2000d).

Except for some advocates at the WHO and UNAIDS, the majority of donors and international organizations considered the provision of ARVs in developing countries unrealistic. The first objection was cost. The provision of ARVs was not considered cost-effective compared to other health interventions, and many feared that the introduction of expensive HIV treatment into development programs would create endless demand for resources that could not be met (Gellman 2000d).[2] The second objection was that the large-scale provision of ARVs was *technically* infeasible in developing countries due to low levels of education and poor medical and public health infrastructure. Andrew Natsios, head of United States Agency for International Development (USAID), still made this argument very forcefully in *The Boston Globe* in 2001 (Donnelly 2001). In the West, ARVs were almost exclusively in the hands of specialized physicians and nurses. Sophisticated tools like T-cell counts were considered indispensable to state-of-the-art antiretroviral therapy. ARVs also required exceptional patient compliance due to their high toxicity. All of these factors were thought to make antiretroviral treatment on a large scale impracticable in developing countries, where health infrastructure was weak, the density and training of medical personnel was insufficient, and patients were poor and uneducated. It was due to these arguments that WHO's proposal to consider alternative pricing schemes as a way of making ARVs more affordable in developing countries, first put on the table by Jonathan Mann, had failed.[3] A third obstacle was seen in the fact that many developing country governments were denying the presence of AIDS in their countries and were doing little to address the stigma associated with the disease (Daley 1998). High-level political commitment was considered a crucial element in any kind of effective policy response (Nogueira 2002).

But in 1995 and 1996, landmark advances in antiretroviral therapy fundamentally changed this landscape. In 1995, the European-Australian Delta study showed that the combination of AZT with a new type of ARVs called protease inhibitors decreased death rates in AIDS patients by 40 percent compared to AZT alone (Chang 1995; Cooper 1996; Delta Coordinating Committee 2001). In 1996, the results of a Boehringer Ingelheim trial showed that a combination of two existing ARVs with their new drug Nevirapine could even reduce the virus below detectable levels (Smart 1996; "Triple Therapy in Previously Untreated Patients Reduces Viral Load Below Limit of Detection" 1996). For the first time since its emergence, HIV/AIDS was no longer an automatic death sentence. HIV-positive individuals who had been prepared to die within few years could suddenly hope to live to old age. It was hoped that triple therapy would eventually eliminate the virus (Krieger 1998). It seemed for some time as if HIV/AIDS would soon be defeated by science. The 1996 Vancouver AIDS conference took place under the rubric "One World, One Hope" (Dunlap 1996).

But the discovery of triple therapy also made more visible the tremendous gap in access to treatment that existed between the industrialized and developing worlds. If you were HIV positive in Switzerland, Sweden, or the United States, you could expect to live many years with the disease. If you happened to live in South Africa or Uganda, you continued to be sentenced to death. National citizenship, not membership in the human species, seemed to determine whether or not a person would die from AIDS or live with the disease.

This changed the spectrum of defensible policy positions. Illness, health, and medicine are seen as universalizing forces. The mere existence of a treatment for a disease somehow carries a normative force that is not seen for other consumer products. It became increasingly difficult for the public health community to legitimize ongoing HIV/AIDS prevention efforts without also offering treatment—for equity reasons. "Access to treatment" became an official motto in international HIV/AIDS policy circles.

Right at the forefront of the "access" discussions was the price of ARVs. Few issues have sparked as much controversy in the context of globalization. Ever since the pharmaceutical company Burroughs Wellcome brought AZT to the U.S. market in 1987, ARV prices had been the focus of intense political struggles between civil society and a powerful industry.[4] The introduction of an extremely expensive treatment for a rapidly fatal disease affecting large numbers of people placed public attention on the prevailing political economy of pharmaceutical innovation. The revenues of the pharmaceutical industry depend on many different factors, including the size of markets and regulatory environments of the nation in which it operates. Exactly *how much* should a pharmaceutical company be allowed to profit from an essential drug that it brings to the market? The answers to such questions were difficult enough in the context of national politics. Globalization only exacerbated the debates.

As much as these breakthroughs in HIV/AIDS treatment changed the expectations of health practitioners, patients, and activists, they may not have sufficed to trigger the tremendous changes to come. A *New York Times* account of the 1998 Geneva AIDS conference transmits dampened enthusiasm about science's ability to defeat HIV/AIDS (Altman 1998)—the article summarized that some of the new AIDS drugs had failed, all of them had been shown to trigger resistances, and on the vaccine front, the first trial of an HIV/AIDS vaccine had rendered monkeys ill without preventing the disease. Overall, it did not look like there was enough momentum to shift the international AIDS policy paradigm from "prevention" to "treatment."

However, a parallel development in the trade and intellectual property domain helped bring the cost of ARVs to the forefront. In 1998, the South African parliament approved a law with the purpose to make essential medicines more affordable to South Africans (Roberts 1998). The law, called the South African Medicines Act, allowed for compulsory licensing and parallel importing of a variety of patent-protected medicines, including ARVs ("Mr. Gore and the AIDS Drugs" 1999; Sternberg 1999). This was the beginning of an unofficial trade war between the United States and South Africa, which lasted several years and was one of the epicenters of the political struggles over ARVs.

Not surprisingly, the law met strong opposition from the pharmaceutical industry, which saw sudden danger to both its efforts to develop new markets and its efforts to protect traditional ones. The founding, in 1995, of the World Trade Organization (WTO) with its arrangements on intellectual property protection had converted developing countries into potential sites of revenue generation. There were two concerns. First, the South African law could set a precedent for other developing countries, encouraging them to infringe on international trade and intellectual property norms even before they were properly established. Second, and much more worrying, was the fact that the law allowed parallel importing. It raised the fear of re-imports of ARVs (and other drugs) from South Africa to North America, Europe, and Japan, where the majority of the industry's revenue was being generated (Gellman 2000d).[5]

The industry had to respond on the national level. The South African Medicines Act was not illegal by international law—according to the rules agreed upon at the founding of the WTO in 1995, developing countries were only required to institute intellectual property rights by 2005 (Gellman 2000d). But the South African Pharmaceutical Trade Group, backed by 40 international pharmaceutical companies, challenged the constitutionality of the law in South African courts (Forman 2008). What looked like a national-level lawsuit quickly came to be seen as an unofficial and hushed trade conflict between South Africa and the United States (see, for example, Sternberg 1999), in which the Clinton administration, lead by Vice President Al Gore, supported the position of the powerful U.S.-based pharmaceutical companies ("Mr. Gore and the AIDS Drugs" 1999). U.S.-based civil society groups started attacking the administration and especially Gore with printed "blood money" and with slogans like "Gore's greed kills" (Gellman 2000a).

In this way, trade integration and the AIDS epidemic, which were unfolding as part of some of the same processes of globalization, collided on one single item: the prices of AIDS drugs. A unique "biopolitical" constellation took shape that provided the basis for political struggles between a wide variety of actors, including a powerful multinational industry, the U.S. government, and an increasingly effective transnational civil society. All of this action was set in South Africa, the country with the highest rate of HIV infection in the world, and marked by the history of racial discrimination in the context of colonial rule. The plight of the poor was effectively pitched against the profits of the rich.

At the eye of the storm were the battles between the industry and the civil society. On one side were critics of the pharmaceutical industry who held the industry responsible for withholding a treatment that could save millions. According to Gellman's account, they included both U.S. and foreign networks and organizations operating at the national and international levels—for example, the U.S. Consumer Project for Technology (CPT) led by James Love, the France-based internationally operating NGO Medecins sans Frontieres (MSF) under the lead of Bernard Pecoul, and the U.S. AIDS Coalition to Unleash Power (ACT UP) in Philadelphia (Gellman 2000a, 2000c). Given the circumstances, this argument said that it was unethical for the industry to be wanting to uphold the rules that govern innovation in modern capitalist societies, because such a policy came at the expense of millions of poor patients in developing countries.

On the other side was the pharmaceutical industry, officially backed by the U.S. government, arguing that the high prices were justified. Moreover, the industry argued that the real obstacles to the provision of antiretroviral medicines in developing countries was not their price but the social, managerial, and political conditions and weak health care infrastructures in these nations (Gellman 2000c). In other words, this argument held that it was the nation-state's responsibility to build the institutional structures that would enable its citizens to access products of pharmaceutical innovation at the price set by the markets.

Finally, there was the international scientific and public health establishment. Some at the WHO and UNAIDS were attempting to negotiate deals on ARV prices with the pharmaceutical companies (see, for example, Gellman 2000d). Other voices were increasingly questioning the industry's argument. *The New England Journal of Medicine's* editor-in-chief, Marcia Angell, published an editorial arguing that given the industry made products of "vital importance to the public health," it should be accountable to "society at large" and not just its own shareholders (Angell 1997). And an increasing number of national and international voices argued that no matter how prices for medicines were determined in the general case, special arrangements were justified in the case of the HIV/AIDS epidemic. International public health experts agreed with South African Health Minister Dlamini-Zuma, who held that HIV/AIDS was as an international emergency that should take precedence over matters of intellectual property (Sternberg 1999).

Hidden behind these controversies about patents and prices was, of course, a much larger issue: who had the responsibility for making antiretroviral treatment accessible to patients in developing countries? Was it the wealthy pharmaceutical industry? Was it the chimerical international community? Was it the rich nations in Europe and the United States? Or was it the governments of HIV/AIDS-affected developing countries? However, for the moment, the focus was on prices.

Clinical Trials

In 1998, a second scientific discovery further changed the range of practicable policy choices—the finding that a short course of AZT combined with delivery by Cesarean section could significantly reduce the probability of mother-to-child transmission of HIV to less than 5 percent (Mandelbrot et al. 1998; The European Mode of Delivery Collaboration 1999). This was a significant improvement over previous results achieved with AZT alone, which reduced the probability of transmission by about two-thirds (Connor, Sperling, and Gelber 1994). It dramatically changed the cost-effectiveness logic of ARVs, at least for one particular segment of an afflicted population: the unborn child. A tool had just become available to dramatically reduce the number of babies infected at birth with a time-limited course of ARVs at controllable cost. Arguing against the provision of ARVs in developing countries suddenly implied not only forsaking millions of adult individuals but also denying millions of newborns the protection from HIV infection at birth. With this information becoming part of the global body of scientific knowledge about HIV/AIDS, a connecting thread had been created among the three globalizing forces of science, trade, and civil society: the issue of mother-to-child transmission of HIV.

The soon-to-be born child has a special claim on the human imagination. It is "concrete" and "local" in that it resides inside the mother's body. Yet at the same time, it also has "abstract" and "global" qualities, as the bearer of life itself. Pregnancy and birth occupy a place of importance in all cultures. Moreover, the newborn child has no agency of its own, and can therefore not be blamed for engaging in risky behavior; it cannot be considered "guilty" of any misfortunes that it is subjected to. As such, it is the epitome of the "innocent victim" of HIV/AIDS. The "sympathetic victim" of HIV/AIDS, whose absence Duff Gillespie previously lamented (Gellman 2000b), had literally been born.

It is therefore not surprising that the fate of the children of HIV-positive mothers and their children had been capturing the international science and public health establishment for a while. And ever since the ACTG076 study showed, in 1994, that AZT can reduce transmission of HIV (Connor, Sperling, and Gelber 1994), a branch of international clinical trials had emerged through which cheaper alternatives were investigated for developing countries; these included shorter courses of AZT, vitamin A, intrapartum vaginal washing, and HIV immune globulin (Lurie and Wolfe 1997). Public health and medicine are normative fields. They seek knowledge to improve treatments for patients. In a very pragmatic move, international HIV/AIDS researchers thus built the high cost of antiretroviral medicines into their research as a variable to be manipulated, like a fact of nature.

It was in the context of these internationally conducted clinical trials that the issue of access to antiretroviral treatment was made in a tangible way involving patients, doctors, and drugs. In the 1980s, patients in developing countries were called on to participate in clinical studies investigating therapies for HIV/AIDS, as part of a tacit norm according to which those affected in any part of the world would help generate scientific knowledge about their disease (see, for example, Perlez 1988). However, in sub-Saharan Africa, the participation in the search for such therapies evidently did not translate into automatic access to such therapies.

In 1997, an article in the *New England Journal of Medicine* claimed that a number of current HIV/AIDS clinical trials in developing countries were unethical because they used placebo groups (Lurie and Wolfe 1997). The World Medical Association's 1964 Declaration of Helsinki on the ethics of clinical trials clearly states that the comparison of a potential treatment with a placebo is ethical only when no effective treatment exists (World Medical Association 1964). In the industrialized world, new treatments are therefore tested against the current standard of care, which in this case would have been AZT, given the results of the ACTG076 study. Yet, as Lurie and Wolfe argued in their article, of 18 trials investigating new ways to prevent the mother-to-child transmission of HIV, all initiated after the completion of ACTG076, only three provided access to AZT to the study participants (two of these were taking place in the United States); the others, which included a total of 17,000 women in several Asian and African countries, all tested their new interventions against placebo (Lurie and Wolfe 1997).

The ensuing controversy revealed a troubling acceptance by the international research community that differences between treatment standards for rich and poor patients are acceptable. All of the studies had been approved by research and ethics councils in the United States and at national and local levels, and involved, either as funders or as implementers, such internationally renowned places as the U.S. National Institutes of Health and Harvard University (Lurie and Wolfe 1997). The authors reasoned that investigators considered the use of placebo justified because "no treatment" (equivalent to the use of placebo) was the standard of care in developing countries and because a design involving placebo controls would make the trials more rapid. They also pointed out that this stance even complied with current thinking at the WHO: in 1994, the WHO had convened an expert group to debate the best research design to investigate cheaper alternatives for the prevention of

AIDS transmission to newborns in developing countries, given the urgency of such research; this group had concluded that placebo-controlled trials offered the best option (World Health Organization 1994; Lurie and Wolfe 1997).

Lurie and Wolfe exposed this implicit double standard and took issue with it, arguing that the ethical standard for the conduct of clinical trials should be universal and that economic reasons could not justify the difference in standards that the use of placebo implied. Their work triggered a controversy among experts that was fought out in some of the world's leading scientific journals. Some agreed. In an influential editorial preceding Lurie and Wolfe's article, the *New England Journal of Medicine*'s editor-in-chief Marcia Angell compared the situation to the infamous Tuskegee Study of Untreated Syphilis in American black men (Angell 1997). In that trial, which took place in the town of Tuskegee, Alabama, U.S. physicians followed a group of male African American syphilis patients for four decades, between 1932 and 1972; they continued to observe the untreated course of the disease even after a cure (penicillin) had become available in 1947 (see Schuman et al. 1955). Others disagreed, making the case that the use of placebo in these cases was justifiable—not because double standards in ethics were inherently defensible, but because the world needed to be pragmatic about finding solutions quickly. Thus, the *British Medical Journal* printed an article written by a team of HIV/AIDS clinicians from South Africa, which argued that while short-course antiretroviral treatment at birth "may be effective," it "shouldn't be allowed to strangle research that might help Africans" (Perinatal HIV Intervention Research in Developing Countries Workshop Participants). The renowned Elizabeth Glaser Pediatric AIDS Foundation and the Emory/Atlanta Center for AIDS Research convened a workshop of leading U.S. HIV/AIDS research organizations explicitly to discuss the topic. Their consensus statement, printed in *The Lancet,* stated carefully that "there are circumstances in which a no-antiretroviral comparison may be ethically justified" (Perinatal HIV Intervention Research in Developing Countries Workshop Participants).

While this controversy took place among experts in the specific context of international clinical trials, the underlying issue was about applicable norms and standards of care in the emerging global health domain. As discussed earlier in text, the fact that ARVs existed in principle was already widely used to argue that they should be *provided* to all HIV/AIDS patients, regardless of their geographical location. However, until the clinical trials controversy, no one had argued that ARVs were being *actively withheld* from patients in developing countries. This changed with the publication of the 1997 article by Lurie and Wolfe. In their view, by conducting clinical trials in developing countries and thereby being physically present in these countries, the international researchers had become *active withholders* of antiretroviral therapy. The article also made visible and explicit the fact that the international community had factored the cost of ARVs into their research logic.

This active withholding of an existing therapy on grounds of race, class, or economic status is precisely what the Tuskegee study notoriously symbolized in the United States. In that study, clinical trials physicians had actively withheld a cure (penicillin) that was available within the geographic boundaries of the United States from a group of African American syphilis patients. Marcia Angell was transporting this reasoning from the national to the global context. In her argument, Tuskegee was now happening globally. National boundaries did not matter, she argued, in determining the ethics of clinical research; the nationalities and economic realities of the patients involved in these trials should play no part in justifying disparate ethical norms in global public health research.

"The Thin End of the Wedge": Saving the Unborn

Of course, the dispute over the design of international clinical trials, however significant, did nothing immediate to change the plight of HIV-positive mothers and their babies in developing countries. In 1998, another controversy erupted, this time over the transmission of HIV during breast-feeding. In searching for ways to reduce the number of HIV-infected babies, the WHO had made the recommendation that HIV-positive women in developing countries feed their babies formula instead of breast-feeding them (Specter 1998). This resulted in an outrage in the development community. Given the lack of clean drinking water in many regions, many regarded the recommendation as plain foolish (Specter 1998). The controversy echoed a previous conflict over the business practices of the Swiss food producer Nestle in the late 1970s and 1980s during which civil society groups claimed that Nestle was "killing babies" by promoting formula in developing countries where there was no stable access to clean water (Gellman 2000c). In *The New York Times,* a Ugandan physician was quoted as saying:

> Twenty-seven percent of babies born to infected mothers become infected from breast-feeding. In rural areas 85 percent of babies will die from dirty water used in formula. I know what they are trying to do, and I applaud the effort. But you don't need a medical degree to figure out which of those odds to take.
>
> (Specter 1998)

Another health official said:

> Is it ethical to bring a baby into this world in that way? Nobody will ever answer that question. We certainly are not going to stop people from having babies.

And it's wonderful that there are ways to treat those children and protect them. But let's not look at formula or a few AZT pills as an answer. It's really just a question. Do women who don't breast-feed want to bring orphans into this world? Or do they want to risk killing their children by caring for them? We're used to death around here. But this is a choice only Idi Amin could have made.

(Specter 1998)

The quotes illustrate the unique political force of the issue of mother-to-child transmission of HIV. The image of Idi Amin, Uganda's inhumane dictator who had sanctioned indescribable cruelties for his private amusement ("Former Ugandan dictator Idi Amin dies" 2003), is invoked here to highlight the inhumanity and waste of human lives caused by the HIV/AIDS epidemic. Thus, these speakers seem to be saying that the situation of HIV-positive mothers is a universal problem, demanding universal treatment by the public health community, even in regions where death of a child has come to be accepted as a normal part of the human condition. Activists and public health officials were referring to the problem as "bitter deaths" (Gellman 2000a), implying that the dying of an HIV-infected baby is not adequately described by the word "death," but needs a suffix, a qualification, to capture what it denotes.

The quotes also illustrate how the representation of HIV/AIDS in purely biomedical terms was perceived as inadequate. HIV/AIDS is presented as a problem that transcends the question of whether or not a virus is transmitted at a particular point during pregnancy and child rearing. If an infant could be protected from infection at birth, and during breast-feeding, what would happen afterward? Would the child then just be orphaned after the mother died of AIDS?

Meanwhile, the pharmaceutical industry was coming under increasing pressure for the prices of its HIV/AIDS treatments. Slogans like "Pfizer's Greed Kills," "Death Under Patent," and "Medical Apartheid" systematically undermined the industry's positioning as a business that merely helps people to be healthy (see Gellman 2000c). At the same time, multilateral organizations were becoming more vocal in their stance on patents and medicines, issuing recommendations that supported the position of developing country governments (Gellman 2000d). Thus, on January 27, 1998, the WHO had issued a revised drug strategy that gave primacy to public health over commercial interests in the case of essential medicines (see, for example, World Health Organization 1998a); earlier, a WHO paper on "Globalization and Access to Drugs" had reviewed the implications of TRIPS (trade-related aspects of intellectual property rights) for public health, stating, "the commercial interests of pharmaceutical corporations can complement public health goals. But just as importantly, they can conflict" and "national governments must maintain the ability to regulate trade in the public interest" (World Health Organization 1997).

In March 1998, after another round of negotiations between UNAIDS and the pharmaceutical industry had failed,[6] there was the first sign of movement on prices. After negotiations with UNAIDS, Glaxo Wellcome announced that it would make AIDS drugs available at prices "substantially below Western market levels" (Gellman 2000d) and would cut down the price of AZT by 75 percent to make it available to pregnant women ("AIDS Drug Cost to Be Cut for Poor Women" 1998; Knox 1998). As a memorandum of the UK Department for International Development phrased it, the mother-to-child transmission of HIV had become "the ethical lightning [rod] of international discussions on drugs access" (see Gellman 2000d). Newborns were the exception from the rule: the one special population to which no one was ready to apply a harsh reality that was true for all other HIV/AIDS patients, namely, that therapy depended on their nationality and economic means. The world was still far from claiming that all HIV/AIDS patients should have access to treatment. Yet as Gellman argues, this was a first step, a fine crack in the wall that stood between patients and their treatment. And civil society and public health groups were well aware of the implications of their victory. As a member of the South African Treatment Action Campaign (TAC) put it to *The Boston Globe*:

> This is the thin end of the wedge. It gives advocacy groups an opening to push for deep discounts on drugs to treat infected people in the developing world.
>
> (Knox 1998)

All Politics Is Local: The Clinton Administration and the Prices of ARVs

Civil society was advancing with respect to the ongoing U.S.—South African trade dispute, too. Gellman describes the evolution, by 1999, of a fierce interagency battle inside the U.S. administration over pharmaceuticals prices in general and the South African lawsuit in particular. One side, led by the U.S. trade office, wanted to escalate the ongoing trade dispute by putting South Africa on the "priority watch list," an act close to formal sanctions as it has the potential to signal a negative environment to investors (Gellman 2000a). The opposition, now led by Al Gore and his chief foreign policy advisor, Leon Fuerth, was concerned about the implications of high ARV prices for countries with severe AIDS epidemics and wanted to find a solution. Gore, who had stopped supporting the pharmaceutical industry after he failed to resolve the trade conflict with South Africa, allied with National Security Council staff and health authorities to block the proposal (Gellman 2000a). In June 1999, Fuerth's office presented a settlement to trade representative Charlene Barshevsky proposing that the United States would withdraw its objections to the South African Medicines Act if South Africa reaffirmed its commitment to as yet unratified patent laws (Gellman 2000a). The apparent reasoning behind this was that if South Africa committed overall to respecting intellectual property according to the WTO model, an end could be put to the dispute.

According to Gellman, the controversy was resolved as a consequence of U.S. civil society pressure on the Gore campaign. He describes that when Al Gore announced his candidacy for the presidency in Carthage, Tennessee, on June 16, 1999, AIDS activists, who had been harassing Gore with the theme of "medical apartheid," were present in the crowd (Gellman 2000a). Partly as a result of the mounting pressure, the Gore campaign connected with AIDS Coalition to Unleash Power (ACT-UP); in the aftermath, Barshefsky signed the settlement proposal, and a few months later, in December, President Clinton announced a new trade policy "flexible enough" so that "people in the poorest countries won't have to go without medicine they so desperately need" (see Gellman 2000c).

Thus, transnational civil society had managed to connect and intertwine two fundamentally national events—a lawsuit against industry in South African courts and Al Gore's candidacy for the American presidency—to advance their claim that access to ARVs should recognize no national boundaries. As was the case during the ethics debate on clinical trials, we find a translation of formerly national discourse to the global level. The term "medical apartheid" not only reflected the fact that the trade dispute had been taking place in South Africa, but also suggested that the crimes of the white race against the black, institutionalized in South Africa's notorious policy of "apartheid," was now being applied on the global level in the form of discriminatory drug prices and treatment standards. Thus, what the invocation of "Tuskegee" did for the special case of clinical trials, the invocation of "apartheid" did for the general case—to establish that the difference in treatment standards due to economic factors was indefensible in the face of the devastation caused by HIV/AIDS.

Evidently, significant changes had taken place by this point in time. The U.S. government and the pharmaceutical industry had made important concessions with respect to the trade dispute; the industry had also offered cheaper drugs for pregnant women. However, the situation was still far from a global commitment to treat all HIV/AIDS patients. Rather, the world had acknowledged a tragedy was ongoing, but was not promising to step in. For this step to happen, a yet another kind of framing was required—HIV/AIDS needed to be seen as a matter that threatens the entire world.

Security Concerns

In 1999 and 2000, important political changes led to a reframing of HIV/AIDS as a global security problem. The year 1999 marked a turning point in the political commitment of African political leaders with respect to HIV/AIDS. It had taken long for African heads of state to acknowledge the problem (with the exception of Zambia's Kenneth Kaunda, who first spoke about HIV/AIDS in 1988) (Altman 1999). The reasons for this reluctance arguable ranged from considerations of national pride to the fear that admitting the existence of HIV/AIDS was going to have repercussions on trade and tourism. On World AIDS Day in December 1998, Nelson Mandela had taken the lead by stating, "it's the silence that is letting this disease sweep through the country. It is time to break the silence" (Altman 1999). Now, after years of insistence by scientists, the WHO, UNAIDS, and other international actors, governments were coming around. At their annual meeting in Addis Ababa, African finance ministers for the first time openly spoke about AIDS, calling it a threat to Africa's economic and social development (Altman 1999).

In January 2000, the UN Security Council devoted an entire session to AIDS ("Action on AIDS in Africa" 2000). For reasons that were hard to explain even for insiders (Gellman 2000b), the Clinton administration, which had the presidency of the Council that year, had completely turned around its approach to HIV/AIDS. Gellman reports about U.S. ambassador to the United Nations, Richard Holbrooke, speaking about the choice of the theme in an interview: "It occurred to me we were going to have the presidency of the Security Council in January, the first month of the millennium. We needed a theme"; Holbrooke also invited Al Gore to present American concerns about this problem (Gellman 2000b). AIDS seemed to be an adequate theme for humanity's entry into the third millennium.

It was a landmark event, the first time that the UN Security Council devoted a meeting to a public health issue. The shorthand version of the Council's conclusions, promptly transported in the press, was that global security would be threatened unless AIDS was controlled in Africa (see, for example, "Action on AIDS in Africa" 2000; Kenna 2000). The spread of AIDS in Africa was declared to be "the worst infectious disease catastrophe since the bubonic plague" ("Action on AIDS in Africa" 2000). As Peter Piot pointed out in an article in *Science* the following June, by defining HIV/AIDS as a human security issue, the Council was understanding human security "not just as the presence or absence of armed conflict" (Piot 2000). During the meeting, world leaders positioned HIV/AIDS as a threat to the fabric of societies certain to undermine past gains in economic development, education, and political stability. To be sure, the comparison to armed conflict figured powerfully in this new image of HIV/AIDS. Thus, Kofi Annan stated that HIV/AIDS killed more human beings than armed conflict in the region, and Al Gore even likened its projected deadly impact in the first decade of the new millennium to "all the wars in all the decades of the twentieth century" (Kenna 2000).

We reencounter in this context the children of HIV-positive parents who figured so importantly in previous discussions about treatment standards. These "innocent victims" of HIV infection at birth and during breast-feeding were now recast as the engine of a global security nightmare:

> Imagine 40 million hungry and destitute orphans in sub-Saharan Africa by the year 2010—roaming the streets without schooling or work, prime candidates for the criminal gangs, marauding militias and child armies that have slaughtered and mutilated tens of thousands of civilians in countries like Sierra Leone and Liberia in the last decade. This is the kind of nightmare that prompted the United Nations Security Council to convene yesterday for an examination of a health issue—the global spread of AIDS, especially in sub-Saharan Africa, where experts predict that more people will die of AIDS in the next decade than have died in all the wars of the 20th century.
>
> ("Action on AIDS in Africa" 2000)

This framing of HIV/AIDS sent a political signal at the highest level. It made a direct connection between HIV/AIDS in Africa and the industrialized world. In this new view, HIV affected not only those who carry it, but *all* human beings, regardless of their HIV status and regardless of which country they happened to be in. Correspondingly, the "public" who was in need of protection from HIV/AIDS was now the whole world. This reframing of HIV/AIDS paved the way for the subsequent redefinition of responsibilities for public health action at the supranational level. The entire world was called upon to act on AIDS, not only for moral reasons but also for reasons of global security. The significance of this reframing was very clear in policy circles. As Peter Piot wrote in *Science:* "Whether we conceptualize AIDS as a health issue only or as a development and human security issue is not just an academic exercise. It defines how we respond to the epidemic, how much money is allocated to combating it, and what sectors of government are involved in the response" (Piot 2000).

Of course, the political signal was only that: a signal. Its most immediate effect was to draw attention to the fact that the resources needed to avert the kind of global security nightmare that was being imagined went far beyond what the international community was spending to fight HIV/AIDS at the time. In 1997, a total of US$ 165 million was devoted on international AIDS prevention, of which only US$ 15 million was used by African governments (Altman 1999). In 1998, that amount rose to about US$ 300 million in development funding, of which UNAIDS accounted for US$ 60 million in annual budget (Piot 2000). At the time, the price of a full course of antiretroviral treatment still stood at US$ 15,000–22,500 per patient per year (Schiller 2000).

Not surprisingly, the question of resources figured prominently in the news coverage of the Security Council meeting. Al Gore announced the United States would add US$ 100 million to its current US$ 225 million spending to fight AIDS overseas (Kenna 2000). However, such promises were in stark contrast to the "global security crisis" rhetoric, and arguably just helped to make the resource gap more visible. *The New York Times* pointed out that the United States was spending US$ 7 billion on the prevention and treatment of HIV/AIDS in the United States alone, where only about 40,000 people were infected ("Action on AIDS in Africa" 2000). Peter Piot stated that at least US$ 1 billion would be needed and pointed out that the resources the West spent on HIV/AIDS in 1997 would "buy less than 12 kilometers of four-lane highway—less than the cost of a single jumbo jet" (Kenna 2000). Zimbabwean Health Minister Timothy Stamps noted that the United States had spent US$ 600 billion just to prevent the Y2K problem (Kenna 2000), which turned out in the end to be a nonproblem. Raising the rhetorical stakes, Stamps accused the West of racial bias because it barred lower-cost generic versions of AIDS drugs that could save millions in Africa, and even asked whether this was "another form of ethnic cleansing" (Kenna 2000). However, no one was promising to pay. For the moment, there was only the statement that HIV/AIDS needed to be addressed at the global level.

Partial Concessions

In March 2000, another controversy erupted over an international HIV/AIDS clinical trial. In a study in the *New England Journal of Medicine,* American researchers reported on the interrelation between sexually transmitted infections and HIV (Quinn et al. 2000). The study, that had been conducted in rural Uganda, was controversial for a number of reasons. First, while all participants were informed of their HIV status, nobody was offered treatment with ARVs. Second, of the patients who were ill with sexually transmitted infections other than HIV/AIDS, only the treatment arm received antibiotics for their infection; the patients in the control arm control group were only informed about the diagnosis and advised to get treated, but not offered treatment. Finally, a subanalysis of the study retrospectively observed how many healthy partners of HIV-positive individuals contracted the virus over the time of the study (Quinn et al. 2000).[7] But as was the case for the clinical studies reported by Lurie and Wolfe earlier, the trial's design had been approved by the review boards of a whole series of preeminent governmental and academic research institutions—thus, as the authors explained in the article, "the AIDS Research Subcommittee of the Uganda National Council for Science and Technology, the human-subjects review boards of Columbia University and Johns Hopkins University, and the National Institutes of Health Office for Protection from Research Risk" had all reviewed the design and had apparently found it to be compliant with their standards and principles (Quinn et al. 2000).

The study was published along with a widely noted editorial by Marcia Angell, in which she expressed doubt about her decision to go ahead with the publication, together with deep concern about the design of the study (Angell 2000). First, she criticized the study for simply observing HIV and STD patients without treating them; second, she took issue with the fact that it observed the frequency of a preventable outcome, the HIV infection of the patients' sexual partners (Angell 2000). Both of these design characteristics, she argued, were impermissible given that an effective treatment for HIV/AIDS existed, and would never have been accepted in a U.S. study. In the editorial, she also directly addressed the question of what role the cost of a therapy should play in the logic that drives research in developing countries:

> Does it matter whether the illness studied is difficult or expensive to treat? Treating HIV infection in rural Uganda would indeed be both difficult and expensive, and at best, the treatment would only stave off AIDS for the duration of the study, not prevent it altogether ... If the expense of antiretroviral therapy justifies not offering it to subjects in certain parts of the world, should that expense be accepted as immutable? Or should we look more closely at the pricing decisions of the manufacturers of drugs protected by patents and the possibility of competition from generic drugs in developing countries.
>
> (Angell 2000)

Shortly thereafter, several things happened with respect to prices. In May 2000, President Clinton issued an order that explicitly communicated that the United States would not interfere with perceived infringements on American patent laws in the African region if they concerned AIDS drugs (Lewis 2000). And within days of this order, five of the world's large pharmaceutical companies—Boehringer Ingelheim, Bristol-Myers Squibb, GlaxoSmithKline, Merck & Co., and Hoffman-LaRoche—and later Abbott Laboratories, with backing from WHO and UNAIDS, announced a reduction of 85–90 percent in the price of AIDS drugs for the developing world (Schiller 2000; see also World Health Organization & Joint United Nations Programme on AIDS 2002).

According to Gellman, this initiative, also called the "Accelerating Access Initiative" (World Health Organization & Joint United Nations Programme on AIDS 2002), was the result of several years of negotiation between the companies and WHO/UNAIDS. He reports that the companies wanted a number of things in return, including a declaration of political commitment to fighting HIV/AIDS on the part of national governments, the build-up of infrastructures and adequate distribution systems necessary to treat HIV/AIDS, an assignment of responsibility for addressing HIV/AIDS to all sectors of society, and finally, an official enforcement of patent rights; in particular, they wanted WHO and UNAIDS to renounce compulsory licensing and parallel importing of drugs (Gellman 2000c). Clearly, they were making the point that cheap drugs alone were not going to achieve the goal of treating patients and that national governments were the main party on whom the responsibility for these patients fell.

The initiative was received with mixed reactions. The WHO and the UN were dissatisfied with the proposal because it did not actually announce a concrete price; African governments felt that the proposal made it appear as though AIDS treatment was now available when it was in reality still out of reach for most developing country health budgets (Gellman 2000c).

Science Versus the Nation-State: Mbeki and the "AIDS Denialists"

In July 2000, the 13th International AIDS Conference took place in Durban, South Africa. Its main theme, "Breaking the Silence," indicated its purpose to fight the lack of governmental openness and political commitment still present in many countries affected by the disease.

The choice of the conference location was no coincidence. For the first time since the emergence of HIV/AIDS, the International AIDS Conference took place not in the West but in a developing country, in an attempt to recognize the burden of AIDS in Africa and to bring science and advocacy to the region (Chaisson 2000). Moreover, South Africa was the country with the largest population of HIV-infected individuals in the world, 4.2 million at the time (Swarns and Altman 2000a). Although the nation with the fastest-growing epidemic, with rates that had risen from 13 to 20 percent in the previous two years ("AIDS in South Africa" 2000), it was also regarded as comparatively well equipped to respond, at least compared to many of its poorer neighbors in the region ("AIDS in South Africa" 2000).

But Durban was to become symbolic in ways that no one had foreseen. In 1999 and 2000, the South African government came under increasing criticism for the way it dealt with HIV/AIDS. Again, the soon-to-be-born child was at the forefront of political struggles. About six months earlier, in 1999, a heated controversy had arisen over the government's refusal to make AZT available to HIV-positive pregnant women in public clinics. The country's president, Thabo Mbeki, and health minister, Manto Tshabalala-Msimang, publicly stated that AZT was too toxic and too expensive to justify its use (Swarns 1999; Goldyn 2000; "In Debate on AIDS, South Africa's Leaders Defend Mavericks" 2000). This enraged many in the public health and advocacy community, who suspected that hidden behind the "toxicity" argument were considerations of cost (James 2000).[8] In addition to this, the fact that US$ 6.2 million of US$ 17 million South African AIDS budget had remained unspent in 1999 ("AIDS in South Africa" 2000; Swarns 2000a) suggested a general "nonchalance" on the part of the government before the country's growing problem.

To complicate matters even more, a further controversy took shape in the months leading up to the Durban conference that was eventually to pitch the South African head of state against the international scientific establishment. It erupted when President Thabo Mbeki invited Peter Duesberg and David Rasnick, two American scientists known to question the link between HIV and AIDS, to be part of a national expert panel he had convened for advice on how best to address HIV/AIDS in South Africa ("In Debate on AIDS, South Africa's Leaders Defend Mavericks" 2000; Swarns 2000a, 2000d). The majority of Mbeki's panel consisted of scientists who affirmed the connection between HIV and AIDS, including the French co-discoverer of HIV, Luc Montagnier (*Presidential AIDS Advisory Panel Report* 2001). But the inclusion of the so-called AIDS denialists prompted a storm of criticism from scientists and nonscientists alike. Mbeki was accused by eminent scientists of investing precious time in evaluating outdated concepts of HIV/AIDS while his country was sliding into a grave situation; some even called for a boycott of the Durban AIDS conference (Swarns 2000c).

The outrage was so great that Mbeki apparently felt the need to explain himself to the world. He sent a letter to President Clinton, UN Secretary-General Kofi Annan, and other world leaders, which was later leaked to *The Washington Post* (Daley 2000; "In Debate on AIDS, South Africa's Leaders Defend Mavericks" 2000; Swarns 2000c). According to contemporary accounts, the letter was so unusual in style that officials in Washington, upon receiving it, initially took it for a "hoax" (Daley 2000). In it, Mbeki talked about his personal journey in grappling with the issue of AIDS and expressed the belief that his country had to find its own specific solution to it, different from the strategies proposed by the West:

> It is obvious that whatever lessons we have to and may draw from the West about the grave issue of HIV-AIDS, a simple superimposition of Western experience on African reality would be absurd and illogical. I am convinced that our urgent task is to respond to the specific threat that faces us as Africans. We will not eschew this obligation in favour of the comfort of the recitation of a catechism that may very well be a correct response to the specific manifestation of AIDS in the West.
>
> (PBS News 2000)

This different African approach, Mbeki was arguing, included the admission of all possibilities and voices, even those that questioned the link between HIV and AIDS.

Deeply frustrated by the reactions of the international community, whom he saw as "tyrannical" and forbidding dissent, Mbeki compared the practices of the scientific establishment with that of the apartheid government:

> Our search for these specific and targeted responses is being stridently condemned by some in our country and the rest of the world as constituting a criminal abandonment of the fight against HIV-AIDS . . . It is suggested, for instance, that there are some scientists who are "dangerous and discredited" with whom nobody, including ourselves, should communicate or interact . . . We are now being asked to do precisely the same thing that the racist apartheid tyranny we opposed did, because, it is said, there exists a scientific view that is supported by the majority, against which dissent is prohibited.
>
> (PBS News 2000)

Mbeki's deputy president Jacob Zuma invoked Galileo:

> Suppose we discover, as Galileo did, that the so-called mainstream scientific view is incorrect. Suppose there was even a 1 percent chance that the solution lay elsewhere. As a country we cannot afford to overlook this possibility.
>
> ("In Debate on AIDS, South Africa's Leaders Defend Mavericks" 2000)

This was a direct attack on science, and science reacted as directly. On April 27, 2000, the prestigious scientific journal *Nature* printed an open letter to Thabo Mbeki in which it defended the institutions of science.[9] The letter's main argument was that quite contrary to what Mbeki and Zuma were suggesting, dissent was fundamental to science, and for this reason, science had developed institutions that allowed it to distinguish legitimate from illegitimate dissent. In a direct comparison between the spheres of politics and science, the letter argued that just as "the ballot box, parliamentary debate and constitutional law" were legitimate methods for collective political decision making, the scientific institution of peer review was the legitimate method to separate "valid heresies" from "those that, after close scrutiny, deserve to be placed aside" ("Dear Mr Mbeki . . . " 2000).

When Mbeki sent his original letter to international political leaders, he arguably did not expect to face the open opposition of the world scientific establishment, as represented by its leading journals, in a public dispute about whether or not it was legitimate to question an established scientific theory. Durban almost turned into a show-down between science and politics. In July 2000, right in time for the conference, *Nature* published the so-called Durban Declaration. In this manifesto, 5,000 scientists declared that "the evidence that AIDS is caused by HIV-1 or HIV-2 is clear-cut, exhaustive and unambiguous, meeting the highest standards of science" ("The Durban Declaration" 2000). It was a truly transnational effort at mobilizing "science" across the world and at all levels. As the text explained, the declaration's signatories included "Nobel prizewinners, directors of leading research institutions, scientific academies and medical societies, notably the US National Academy of Sciences, the US Institute of Medicine, Max Planck institutes, the European Molecular Biology Organization, the Pasteur Institute in Paris, the Royal Society of London, the AIDS Society of India and the National Institute of Virology in South Africa," as well as individual scientists from industrialized and developing countries. Scientists at pharmaceutical companies, it was noted, had not been asked to participate. The declaration was thus uniting global public sector science to convince the world that its view of HIV/AIDS was the one to subscribe to, independent of geography. And so were the conclusions that this view implied: "It is unfortunate that a few vocal people continue to deny the evidence. This position will cost countless lives," the declaration said—"in this global emergency, prevention of HIV infection must be our greatest worldwide public-health priority."

South African authorities were quick to stress that Mbeki never explicitly denied the causal relationship between HIV and AIDS (Swarns 2000b). An aggressive HIV/AIDS prevention campaign the South African government was running at the time was based on education about sexual transmission of HIV (Altman 2000b). So what precisely was so heretical about Mbeki's action? Science is a way of representing reality that is considered fundamental to our understanding of the world. By including "AIDS denialists" in his panel, Mbeki was giving voice to those who were seen as "telling the world as it is not." In flirting with the possibility, however remote, that mainstream science was wrong about HIV and AIDS, Mbeki was seen as questioning the scientific representation of HIV/AIDS that allowed humanity to create order from disorder and thereby to seek solutions to grave threats to human well-being. By questioning the scientific representation of AIDS, Mbeki was seen as simultaneously questioning the *solution* embedded in this representation, namely, the idea that the prevention of HIV infection as a large-scale public health measure was the correct strategy for fighting HIV/AIDS everywhere in the world.

Mbeki's letter triggered a second debate, different from the first, yet intimately intertwined with it. This was over the question of whether South Africa had to follow a separate path or whether it should follow the prescriptions of the international public health establishment. This debate had two streams, led by two different groups. Speaking at the Durban conference, Mbeki had singled out "extreme poverty" as the root cause of AIDS: "As I listened and heard the whole story told about our own country, it seemed to me that we could not blame everything on a single virus" (Swarns and Altman 2000a). Some selected this part of Mbeki's argument to explore the notion that while HIV caused AIDS, its epidemiological patterns in Africa were not fully grasped by the current scientific paradigm, which emphasized its viral origins, and potentially needed alternative solutions (see, for example, letters to the editors of *Science* and *Nature* at the time, Markus and Fincham 2000; Oliver 2000).

But others used it to counter the arguments of those who wanted to make ARVs universally available. For them, Mbeki's inviting of Rasnik and Duesberg was merely a detour, however lamentable, on the way to the position that the large-scale provision of ARVs was infeasible in a country like South Africa. A *New York Times* editorial entitled "Africa Can't Just Take a Pill for AIDS" argued:

> Mr. Mbeki[s] ... iconoclasm began to make sense. He focused on a stark reality: the pharmaceutical-based model of H.I.V. care in the West is not applicable to South Africa. He may be arriving at this conclusion by a route involving some indefensible detours, but the conclusion itself is sound... If cheaper drugs arrived in South Africa by the shipload, how would one get people to take them? The history of another disease, tuberculosis, is sadly instructive. For years some southern African nations have had large-scale TB programs with cheap, easy-to-take drugs, but have not made a dent in infection rates.
>
> (Goldyn 2000)

We see in this passage the familiar arguments of opponents of the provision of ARVs at that time. The author, Lawrence Goldyn, argues that the *cost* of ARVs and the *intricacies of their use* justified a "separate African solution," regardless of whether or not one believed in the connection between HIV and AIDS. What looked like a discussion about the biomedical interpretation of HIV and AIDS was really a controversy about a constellation of factors that might be labeled "biopolitical" or "bioeconomical." If a single dose of penicillin had been shown to eliminate HIV quickly and cheaply, very likely none of these controversies would have occurred. Interestingly, in the article, Goldyn finds the case of mother-to-child transmission of HIV "immediately more compelling," a statement that illustrates once more the tremendous political force of this issue. However, he still holds the view that even saving the unborn isn't quite an option given poor infrastructure: "As Mr. Mbeki says, the Western model of fighting AIDS is of little use to Africa now," Goldyn concludes.

To be sure, both universal access to ARVs and Mbeki's stance on HIV/AIDS were at the top of the Durban agenda. South African Supreme Court Justice Edwin Cameron, himself HIV positive, severely criticized the South African government for accusing political leaders of "irresponsibility that borders on criminality" (Chaisson 2000); he also argued that the international community had a responsibility to provide antiretroviral medicines to all HIV/AIDS patients in the world:

> No more than Germans in the Nazi era, no more than white South Africans during apartheid, can we at this conference say that we bear no responsibility for 30 million people in resource poor countries who face death from AIDS unless medical care and treatment is made accessible to them.
>
> (Chaisson 2000)

In Cameron's vision, the "public" whose health needed protection was defined as "30 million people in resource poor countries." By likening the failure to treat HIV/AIDS in developing countries to ethnic cleansing and racist genocide, Cameron was making the same argument that Angell and others had previously made with respect to clinical trials: that *not providing treatment* is the same as *actively withholding treatment*. However, Cameron was going one step further. The physical presence of those who have access to treatment was no longer required to fulfill the condition of "nontreatment" as a political act. Moreover, by extending the examples of national policies of discrimination to the global level, Cameron was arguing that the responsibility to act on HIV/AIDS no longer lay with nation-states alone but with the international community. Peter Piot and others extended Cameron's argument to the whole world, arguing that "billions, not millions" were needed to fight AIDS everywhere: at least US$ 3 billion to provide the most basic set of measures in Africa and an additional tens of billions annually to provide antiretroviral therapy to patients in all developing countries (Swarns and Altman 2000a).

Thus, Durban was the arena in which the proponents and opponents of universal access to ARVs faced each other in a unique way. South Africa was the symbolic and particular location for these struggles. On the one hand, South Africa had withstood all attempts by the U.S. government to pressure it into yielding on the price issue, suggesting support for the proponents' position. On the other hand, Mbeki's flirtation with the AIDS denialists suggested that drugs were not the solution to the nation's AIDS problem.

Generic Competition

In 2001, the prices of ARVs came down dramatically through generic competition. However, at the beginning of that year, the situation was still far from transparent. The Accelerating Access Initiative had prompted a number of separate programs, which were structured as public-private partnerships and usually involved the free provision of drugs to certain countries or patient subgroups. As an example, Merck was cooperating with the Bill and Melinda Gates Foundation and the government in Botswana to provide US$ 100 million for fighting HIV/AIDS, which the press termed a "virtual Marshall plan" (Collins 2000); as part of the plan, Merck was offering to supply its compounds Crixivan and Sustiva for free to Botswanan patients. Similarly, Boehringer Ingelheim was working with a consulting firm to aid the free distribution of its Viramune for the prevention of mother-to-child transmission to programs in Africa (Waldholz 2001). However, while these initiatives were real and important, and notably the Merck initiative has since been viewed as successful (see, for example, Ramiah and Reich 2006), there was no overall coordination on the price of ARVs.

In addition, given the drugs were being given away for free, the companies' interest in participating in joint large-scale ventures to roll out antiretroviral treatment had to be limited. According to Gellman, some executives saw the new activities mainly in the context of efforts to improve the industry's image and, in the long run, unlock new markets—the future of the pharmaceutical industry was seen in markets for adult chronic diseases all over the world, and HIV/AIDS certainly fit right into this concept because ARVs were a means to control, but not cure, the virus (Gellman 2000c). He reports on a Dutch initiative, in which an HIV/AIDS researcher named Joep Lange, who was also a member of Boehringer Ingelheim's scientific advisory board, approached the five companies participating in the Accelerating Access Initiative to see if they would make antiretroviral treatment available at a discounted price for a program to treat 1 million individuals in African countries, financed by their employers—"they laughed at us," Lange reportedly said (Gellman 2000c).

But in September 2001, an offer from the Indian generics company CIPLA suddenly dropped the price of triple therapy to US$ 600 per person per year ("Fighting AIDS in Africa" 2001; McNeil Jr. 2001). The company had already been offering generic triple therapy within India, as the country's domestic intellectual property regime only provided for patents on manufacturing processes (not on the resulting chemical compounds), and India was not obliged to adopt WTO patent rules until 2005 (Gellman 2000c). Now CIPLA was publicly proposing to sell the chemical equivalents of some of the newest antiretroviral agents, including Epivir (lamivudine, produced by Glaxo), Viramune (nevirapine, produced by Boehringer Ingelheim), Zerit (stavudine, produced by Bristol-Myer Squibbs), and Crixivan (indinavir produced by Merck) to UN agencies and international NGOs at manufacturing cost, as a "global public service" (Gellman 2000c).

This was a landmark event. Its most immediate effect was to expose the enormous difference between the price of ARVs and their manufacturing cost. But even more significant was the fact that CIPLA had "gone global": the company was offering ARVs at a single price to multiple actors in the international domain. In that sense, CIPLA's bold move was a daring moment in the history of international pharmaceuticals. In March 2001, the company went a step further: it asked the South African government for a compulsory license for the introduction of triple therapy into the South African market (Swarns 2001g).[10]

Not surprisingly, the pharmaceutical industry's reaction was hostile. It protested against what was seen as piracy (Gellman 2000c). The metaphorical term "piracy" suggests that laws were being violated in a space in which existing laws cannot be enforced, much as actual pirates could not be stopped on the open seas. However, by that time, public opinion had changed. As one observer noted, ARVs had shown a stronger effect on AIDS mortality than penicillin had demonstrated when its efficacy against sepsis was discovered— "now contrast this with the fact that . . . [most patients do not have] access to such treatment, and that you can produce these drugs and can produce them cheaply. You will then start to understand the urgency and indeed the rage behind the clamor for access" (Gellman 2000c). The pharmaceutical industry eventually acquiesced. In March 2001, the large companies gave way: first Merck, then Bristol-Myers Squibb (Petersen and McNeil Jr. 2001), and then Abbot (Petersen 2001). Another norm had changed for HIV/AIDS: that of pharmaceutical companies setting or negotiating the prices of their drugs country by country.

In April 2001, the 39 companies that had sued South Africa in 1998 also officially dropped the ongoing lawsuit, declaring that the South African Medicines Act was not in conflict with international trade law and offering to pay the South African government's legal costs (Swarns 2001d, 2001e). The dispute had come to be seen as the epitome of the pharmaceutical industry's indifference to African suffering ("South Africa's AIDS Victory" 2001). It was a framing the industry could not politically or commercially sustain. "We don't exist in a vacuum," GlaxoSmithKline's CEO Jean-Pierre Garnier told *The New York Times*, admitting that public opinion was an important factor in the company's decision making (Swarns 2001d). "We have never been opposed to wider access. We have discounted our drugs. We've done everything we could. Frankly, the legislation was the worst distraction. It did not allow us to communicate our message effectively," he told the newspaper.

Feasibility: The Renegotiation of Global Aids Treatment Standards

Of course, the sudden drop in the price of ARVs did not directly increase access to antiretroviral treatment for patients in developing countries. Even in relatively well equipped South Africa, where the national Medical Research Council had officially declared AIDS the chief cause of death in October 2001 (Swarns 2001a), antiretroviral therapy became available only after the South African courts ordered the government to make it available to special groups: pregnant women and victims of rape.[11]

Now that HIV/AIDS was established in its status as a global emergency, and antiretroviral therapy had been moved into the realm of affordable interventions, the last remaining conceptual obstacle to universal access came into the focus of discussions. This was the question whether the large-scale provision of antiretroviral treatment in developing countries was technically feasible or not. Donors had two main concerns. First, the lack of personnel and technologies needed for state-of-the-art antiretroviral therapy would make the endeavor impossible; second, the low levels of education of individuals in developing countries would prevent them from correctly adhering to the complicated therapy regimes (Gellman 2000d; Goldyn 2000). In addition, it was argued that the imperfect management of ARV treatment could quickly give rise to drug-resistant strains of HIV emerge, rendering them useless (see, for example, the study by Vergne et al. 2002).

This view was challenged gradually, through scientific proof that adequate treatment was feasible in infrastructure-poor settings. A few dedicated academic teams and NGOs had started to run treatment programs in poor communities to counter these arguments. The French NGO Doctors Without Borders did pioneering work introducing antiretroviral treatment in one of Cape Town's poorest shanty towns, Kayelitsha (Levy, Miksad, and Fein 2005). Based on his earlier experience with tuberculosis treatment in resource-poor settings, Paul Farmer had introduced a community-based ARV treatment program (referred to as "DOT-HAART") in rural Haiti, which was specifically designed to prove that a high-tech environment was not a precondition for effective and professional use of ARVs (see Farmer et al. 2001a, 2001b; Behforouz, Farmer, and Mukherjee 2004). Their approach, as described in these studies, was based on a system in which local lay people were trained as "accompagnateurs" and remunerated for conducting daily visits to HIV patients in their communities, directly supervising and supporting them in taking ARVs. One of their studies, a scale-up to 8,000 rural patients, was also using "low tech," clinical parameters of success, such as weight gain, and the frequency with which opportunistic infections occurred, to monitor treatment success (Koenig, Léandre, and Farmer 2004).

This pilot work functioned as a "proof of principle" that all of the previously mentioned concerns—feasibility, adherence, measurement of effective treatment, and generation of resistances—could be overcome. Farmer and his colleagues had offered the world a peer-reviewed redefinition of what "state of the art" antiretroviral therapy means. Their approach also represented a shift from a "biomedical" framework to one that emphasized social components of health care and medicine. The "technology" that needed scaling up was not the pill itself, but the microlevel institutions built to ensure its regular administration. Farmer made this argument for both the developing and the industrialized world by testing the *accompagnateurs* scheme in both Haiti and Boston. He explained that his Haitian patients were getting better treatment than some of the HIV/AIDS patients with severe exacerbations of their disease he saw in the emergency room at Massachusetts Hospital. Given many of these cases were due to a lack of adherence to the antiretroviral therapy regimens, Farmer argued that the help and encouragement of an *accompagnateur* would help patients comply with and thus substantially improve the outcomes of the therapy.[12]

"Billions, Not Millions": The Road to the Global Fund

Paul Farmer's findings were an important building block in ensuing debates about the feasibility of large-scale antiretroviral treatment programs in developing countries. In March 2001, a group of Harvard academics led by economist Jeffrey Sachs published a widely noted proposal in which they synthesized *ethical, medical, political,* and *economic* reasons for why the international community should urgently address the disparity in access to antiretroviral drugs between developing countries and the industrialized world with adequate resources (Individual Members of the Faculty of Harvard University 2001). Their proposal built on all of the hard-fought conclusions about the relation between HIV/AIDS and human rights, economic development, and human security of the previous years: the argument that ARV therapy was necessary to sustain the plans and strategies developing countries had made for their economic development; the argument that Africa's children needed to be saved from becoming AIDS orphans in order to prevent a global security disaster; the argument that treatment was not only necessary to save millions of HIV infected individuals, but was also an essential part of HIV prevention; and the argument, based on Farmer's work, that antiretroviral therapy was feasible in resource-poor settings (Individual Members of the Faculty of Harvard University 2001).

But most importantly, the proposal set out a concrete financing plan. It estimated that donor aid of US$ 4.2 billion would be needed over the first five years of a global treatment effort (at US$ 1,100 per patient per year), and even suggested where that money might come from: a new funding mechanism set up independent of the United Nations system in order to raise and distribute the resources necessary to finance the operation (Individual Members of the Faculty of Harvard University 2001).

The proposal generated heated discussion in the development community. Andrew Natsios, then director of USAID, famously dismissed the idea of treating Africans with ARVs with the argument that Africans were unable to adhere to complicated treatment regimens because they lacked any (Western) notion of time (Donnelly 2001):

> Many Africans don't know what Western time is. You have to take these (AIDS) drugs a certain number of hours each day, or they don't work. Many people in Africa have never seen a clock or a watch their entire lives. And if you say, one o'clock in the afternoon, they do not know what you are talking about. They know morning, they know noon, they know evening, they know the darkness at night. I'm sorry to be saying these things, but a lot of people like Jeffrey Sachs advocating these things have never worked in health care in rural areas in Africa or even in the cities.

But by the beginning of 2001, thinking in the development community had already shifted and calls for a new funding mechanism for HIV/AIDS had become strong, arising from several sources (see Copson and Salaam 2005). A first proposal by France, at the 1998 G8 summit in Birmingham, for an international funding mechanism to fight AIDS had not generated wide interest (Copson and Salaam 2005, 2). In August 1999, Representative Barbara Lee of California proposed an "AIDS Marshall Plan Fund" to the 106th United States Congress, which proposed a separate U.S. agency run with funding from governments (U.S. and foreign) and from the private sector (Copson and Salaam 2005, 2). In January 2000, Representative

James Leach of Iowa proposed a "Global AIDS and Tuberculosis Relief Act," which contained provisions for a "World Bank AIDS Trust Fund" granting money to developing country governments and NGOs to fight AIDS (Copson and Salaam 2005, 2). In July 2000, the U.S. government had offered Africa US$ 1 billion in loans to pay for AIDS treatment (Kahn 2000).

These proposals are evidence of the new political commitment to address HIV/AIDS. Some proposed loans, other grants with varying national and multilateral institutional affiliations. However, based on the argument that the AIDS epidemic is so overwhelming that traditional foreign aid cannot cover it, these initiatives increasingly arrived at the single conclusion that, instead of traditional models, governments (rich as well as poor) should align with the public and private sectors in an expanded concept of development aid (Crossette 2001). The time seemed ripe not just for a commitment but also for a new approach to aid.

In April 2001, Kofi Annan, during a speech he held at a meeting of the Organization of African Unity in Nigeria, for the first time proposed a "Global Fund" to address AIDS and other infections (Crossette 2001; Copson and Salaam 2005). "The war on AIDS," he explained, "will not be won without a war chest, a size far beyond what is available so far," stating that US$ 7–10 billion will be needed annually (Crossette 2001). Soon after, Annan next presented the idea to a meeting in Philadelphia of wealthy privately owned foundations, expressing to their representatives and the belief that in this age of globalization, an entirely different model of collective action was needed to address a global disease:

> You have understood the nature of our times: an age when the global and the local can no longer be separated; and when governments can no longer tackle global challenges alone. They need new partners . . . In today's world, there are no health sanctuaries—no separation between "foreign" and "domestic" infections; and no "us" and no "them."
>
> (United Nations General Assembly 2001)

Soon after this meeting, first steps were taken on the road toward creating the Global Fund. At a meeting of the G-7 that focused on a larger program for the provision of antiretroviral treatment, James Wolfensohn, president of the World Bank, said an annual US$ 3–4 billion would be needed to construct a reliable program; in comparison, UNAIDS was at the time just approaching US$ 1 billion in annual commitments (Crossette 2001). On May 11 that year, Annan, in the company of Nigerian President Obasanjo, came to the White House, where President George W. Bush made a "founding pledge" of US$ 200 million to the new fund, promising more as the fund went along and stressing the need for the Global Fund to be organized as a public-private partnership (Copson and Salaam 2005). Shortly thereafter, initial talks about a Global Fund began in Washington among the G8 countries.

In June 2001, the United Nations endorsed the creation of a Global Fund. In its first Special Session on a public health issue, the UN General Assembly issued the UNGASS Declaration of Commitment on HIV/AIDS, with three crucial components: first, it recognized access to treatment as a basic need; second, it stated the commitment of the community of nation-states to come up with the needed resources of US$ 7–10 billion annually by 2005 for "prevention, care, treatment, support, mitigation" of HIV/AIDS; third, it recommended the creation of a "global HIV/AIDS and health fund to finance an urgent and expanded response to the epidemic based on an integrated approach to prevention, care, support and treatment" (United Nations General Assembly 2001). The world had officially declared that it was going to financially support the developing world's response to HIV/AIDS.

After this endorsement by the United Nations, the G8 summit in Genoa also endorsed the new fund (which some therefore called the "Genoa Trust Fund") and affirmed that it would be a public-private partnership, operational by the end of 2001 (Copson and Salaam 2005). Shortly thereafter, a "Transitional Working Group" (TWG) was set up. It included government representatives from developing and developed countries, as well as NGOs, UN and private sector representatives, and it had reached, by the end of 2001, agreement on the basic structure of governance and accountability for the Global Fund (see Copson and Salaam 2005). The first Global Fund board meeting was held in January 2002 (Kapp 2002) and in March the Fund announced its first round of funding (Ramsay 2002).

Conclusion

The Global Fund, as I have shown in this chapter, emerged from political struggles over the provision of antiretroviral medicines in developing countries. While the controversies over the prices of antiretroviral medicines were the most visible aspect of these struggles, the redefinition of HIV/AIDS took place at many different levels and included a variety of different actors, including national governments, multilateral organizations, and civil society.

The coming into being of this new organization required a fundamental reframing of the meaning of HIV/AIDS at the global level. HIV/AIDS was redefined from a serious public health problem affecting certain nation-states to a global development and security issue affecting all human beings. This redefinition happened through the three interdependent pathways of science, markets, and civil society action. The issue of mother-to-child transmission of HIV/AIDS served as a connecting thread among these forces.

In the process of the redefinition of HIV/AIDS as a global problem, international standards and norms were challenged in such diverse domains as politics, trade and intellectual property, medicine, and ethics. As a consequence, the responsibilities of existing actors in the health domain were redefined. Before 2002, none of the major players had wanted to commit to taking responsibility for addressing the HIV/AIDS epidemic. Now it had been established that the international community, as represented by the United Nations and the G8 summit, were going to provide resources for the treatment of HIV/AIDS in developing countries through a new funding mechanism established outside the multilateral institutions. For the first time, local actors are now able to access a separate financing mechanism for support in grants (not loans) of their national HIV/AIDS prevention and treatment programs. The institutional realization of this basic principle is the Global Fund.

CHAPTER 4

How the Fund Operates in the Global Domain

This chapter is devoted to the Global Fund as an institution. High hopes are pinned to this new body's ability to make a dent in three important global health issues. In the face of the terrible devastation caused by the HIV/AIDS, tuberculosis, and malaria epidemics, the world has decided to break with the "business as usual" of the socioeconomic divide that keeps the poor South from having access to the same medicines as the wealthy North by making treatment available to all who need it, independent of nationality. To this aim, it has created a new "global" organization, one that would "not belong to one set of countries, or be tied to the United Nations, the World Bank or other institutions," but one that would at the same time be a "genuinely international entity" and a "partnership between the public and private sectors" (World Health Organization 2002a, 1).

But what exactly does that mean? Now that the Fund exists, how does it imagine the global domain and its actors? How does it conceptualize health and disease, global and local, public and private, science and knowledge? What rules does it introduce into the emerging global domain? And how does it gain authority to act in it? In order to answer these questions, I will examine, in this chapter, the Fund's institutional design.

I argue that the Fund at once shapes and is shaped by the scale at which it operates. Co-production regards institutions as society's "inscription devices" (Latour and Woolgar 1979; Latour 1987) or as "vehicles through which the validity of new knowledge can be accredited . . . and accepted rules of behavior written into the as-yet-unordered domains that have become accessible through knowledge-making" (Jasanoff 2004, 40). Viewed from this perspective, the Fund initially emerged as a way of creating order in the disorder of HIV/AIDS. We are thus witnessing the simultaneous emergence of a matter to be governed (global HIV/AIDS, tuberculosis, and malaria) and the tools with which to govern it (the Global Fund). For the purpose of this study, the Global Fund is therefore simultaneously a product of co-production and a vehicle or an agent of co-production—it has rules built into it but also creates and changes rules as it begins its work in the global domain.

In a nutshell, the Fund envisions a new way of conducting development aid. It wants to rearrange the relations between the existing players in such a way that local actors drive the response to HIV/AIDS, tuberculosis, and malaria with financial support—but without interference—from donor countries. Accordingly, it defines roles for a variety of players in the global health domain, including national governments, intergovernmental agencies, companies, nongovernmental organizations, and patients. The Fund itself is situated at the center of these actors, connecting them in new ways and coordinating their interaction across global and local levels according to a specific set of rules.

The rules are defined by the Fund's needs to balance the principle of accountability at two levels. On the one hand, it must keep its promise to empower local actors. On the other hand, it must stay accountable to the donors who provide the funding. As the chapter will show, the fund aims to achieve this by combining a political institution (local stakeholder inclusion) at the local level with a scientific institution (technical review) at the global level. This effectively assigns to "science" the role of judging the validity of local policy. It also conceptualizes science as a set of norms that transcend nation and culture.

The Fund's ability to claim legitimacy and accountability hinges on the way in which it conceptualizes the relation between science and politics in that domain. In the process of defining rules along the two axes of local/global and science/politics, the Fund creates new forms of identity. Three different types of "experts" emerge, each with a particular set of skills that are relevant to the Fund's work. A "global consumer" is also imagined, whose financial contribution to the Fund happens independent of nationality. The conclusion discusses implications of the Fund's vision of global policy making for its work in that domain.

The Fund's Purpose, Scope, and Mission

The 2001 UNGASS meeting established that a new "Global Fund" for AIDS would be set up. Preparations for the setup proceeded amidst lively debates about its exact purpose (see, for example, the *British Medical Journal* editorial by Brugha and Walt 2001). What was the justification to create a new mechanism versus channeling resources through existing systems? And how was the relation between the Fund and other efforts to tackle HIV/AIDS going to be defined? Three major arguments were put forward to justify the creation of a new mechanism. In May 2002, Anders Nordstrom, at the time interim executive director of the Fund, summarized them in a letter to *The Lancet* (see, for example, Nordstrom 2002a): first, a new Fund could catalyze the raising of new financial means more effectively than an existing body; second, it would be able to rapidly disburse these funds and yield visible results on the ground; and third, creating a separate institution for the three diseases would help to increase global attention for them. With respect to the relation between the new organization and other efforts, the Fund was seen as one pillar in a larger approach that would include developed and developing country governments as well as other partners (Nordstrom 2002a, 2002b).

A consultation process was initiated to work out fundamental questions of public health. A first set of questions was related to the Fund's focus and mission. Some were referring to the new organization as the "AIDS Fund" (Hale 2001a), while others called it the "global health fund" (Brugha and Walt 2001; Ford and T'Hoen 2001). Some argued that it should include the major diseases of childhood (see Brugha and Walt 2001) or that it should support the building up of health systems (Brugha and Walt 2001; Lambert and van der Stuyft 2002).

A second set of questions asked which countries should receive money through the Global Fund. Should funding be made available to *all* developing countries or only the poorest countries? And how far should the eligibility for Global Fund monies be determined by the severity of the burden of the three diseases in the respective applicant country? For example, should middle-income countries with low HIV infection rates be equally entitled to Global Fund money as sub-Saharan African countries with infection rates of over 30 percent in their adult population?

Finally, there was the question of which interventions the Fund would support. The idea that offering prevention without simultaneously making treatment available was an unsuccessful way of running HIV/AIDS programs had gained currency among international health policy makers (see, for example, Hale 2001b), and the UNGASS meeting had already declared that antiretroviral treatment *was* going to be part of the new Fund's mission (United Nations General Assembly 2001). However, it was not clear when that would start. Some argued there should be little focus on treatment initially, because "funding HAART at the expense of prevention means greater loss of life" (Marseille, Hofmann, and Kahn 2002); others held that treatment must be a core component of all Global Fund-supported programs from the beginning (Hale 2001b).

The consultation process included representatives from 38 countries (developing as well as developed countries) and organizations (public and private sector organizations).[1] It was set up to define the fundamental features of the Global Fund (World Health Organization 2002a). The committee decided that the Global Fund should be a vertical organization focusing on the three biggest infectious killers in developing countries: HIV/AIDS, tuberculosis, and malaria. However, the strengthening of health systems would also be a central part of its mission.[2]

It was decided that the Global Fund would give "due priority to areas with the greatest burden of disease, while strengthening efforts in areas with growing epidemics" (The Global Fund to Fight Aids, Tuberculosis and Malaria 2002a). The Global Fund framework document specifies a combination of epidemiological, economic, and political criteria for eligibility: the overall burden of disease and the potential for a sudden increase in its incidence and prevalence; the applicant country's poverty level as measured, for example, by GNP per capita or the UN Human Development Index; the level of government commitment to addressing the disease, as measured by the level of government financing for pertinent public health programs, the existence of relevant national policies, and the overall government spending on health (The Global Fund to Fight Aids, Tuberculosis and Malaria 2005b). Treatment was part of the Fund's program starting in round one.

After these basic questions of focus, scope, and mission were worked out, the final and arguably biggest task was that of determining how the Fund should go about allocating its resources. How would responsibilities be distributed in the Fund's system? How were decisions going to be made? And what rules would govern resource allocation through the Fund? Two basic goals emerged in the ensuing discussions about the Fund's governance system. First, there was the call for "a completely new model of aid management" (Richards 2001), a new organization that "makes effective action likely, satisfies donors, responds efficiently, and produces observable results" (Poku 2002). Second, there was the argument that the Fund should follow developing country priorities, not donor priorities (Richards 2001; Yamey and Rankin 2002). As the following section will show, the Fund's institutional design and practices are shaped by its efforts to reconcile these two goals.

Institutional Design

The Global Fund's website tells us that the Fund is "a partnership between governments, civil society, the private sector and affected communities" (The Global Fund to Fight Aids, Tuberculosis and Malaria 2006b). Essential features of its design were already laid out in the 2001 proposal led by Jeffrey Sachs and colleagues, who had initially called for a "single, global HIV/AIDS Prevention and Treatment Trust Fund" under joint WHO and UNAIDS leadership, supported by scientific institutions like the WHO and the U.S. National Institutes for Health (NIH), and funded by donor governments, and who had pronounced the vision for a system in which the initiative for action, the design of a health intervention, and the responsibility for implementation all lie entirely with the applicant country (Individual Members of the Faculty of Harvard University 2001, 16–17). To realize this vision, the Fund introduces a variety of new governance tools at local and global levels.

In this section, I will focus on the rules that govern the interaction between the Global Fund and its recipients. Among the core principles of the Fund's institutional design, four stand out. The first is an emphasis on science and expertise as central to effective public health action:

> There is abundant evidence that science based HIV prevention is effective, especially when backed by high level political leadership, a national AIDS programme, adequate funding, and strong community involvement.
>
> (The Global Fund to Fight Aids, Tuberculosis and Malaria 2008a)

> Over the past three decades, public health experts have identified a number of highly effective interventions to prevent and treat AIDS, TB and malaria. If brought to scale, such efforts could change the course of these diseases. However, achieving this scale-up would require a substantial increase in resources.
>
> (The Global Fund to Fight Aids, Tuberculosis and Malaria 2008b; 2012a, 6)

Suggesting that "science based HIV prevention" must be "backed" by politics assigns a fundamental role to science and expertise.

A second central notion is that of "local ownership," or the idea that the projects it funds are locally initiated, designed, and implemented. The Global Fund invites applications from developing countries in successive "rounds." In most cases, the application will come from a representative of the state, for example, the Ministry of Health or a disease control agency. However, the Fund provides for the possibility that country-level actors submit directly to the Fund (bypassing the government and CCM), in case of countries "without legitimate governments," those "facing conflict or facing natural disasters," and those that "suppress or have not established partnerships with civil society and NGOs" (The Global Fund to Fight Aids, Tuberculosis and Malaria 2002a). Once a grant has been approved, the responsibility for implementation is conceived of as lying entirely with the local actor. Thus, the

Fund does not take an active role in the initiation or implementation of the programs it supports. The Global Fund's website states:

> The Global Fund's purpose is to attract, manage and disburse resources to fight AIDS, TB and malaria. We do not implement programs directly, relying instead on the knowledge of local experts.
>
> (The Global Fund to Fight Aids, Tuberculosis and Malaria 2006b)

A third major pillar of the Fund's institutional design is the concept of stakeholder inclusion in local decision making. A mandated stakeholder inclusion process, called the *Country Coordinating Mechanism* (CCM), serves to ensure that multiple local actors—including civil society and patients—actively take part in health program design. The Fund's guidelines suggest that the CCM be constructed on the basis of a national-level HIV/AIDS committee and requests that it be made up of representatives of government, business, civil society, the academic sector, religious organizations, multi- and bilateral development agencies, and individuals who are affected by the diseases (The Global Fund to Fight Aids, Tuberculosis and Malaria 2005b, 4). Every CCM member needs to approve of the application before it can be submitted to the Fund, and thus has the ability to veto a proposal.

The CCM's main functions are to oversee both the design and submission as well as the implementation of Global Fund-supported programs (The Global Fund to Fight Aids, Tuberculosis and Malaria 2005b, 2). It also determines the *Principal Recipient* (PR) of the grant, which can be a government agency or an NGO that is in charge of implementing the project at the local level (The Global Fund to Fight Aids, Tuberculosis and Malaria 2005b, 2). The CCM is thus a fundamental piece of the Global Fund's architecture, embodying the three principles of local ownership, multisectoral collaboration, and participatory decision making. It is through this institutional structure—a local public-private partnership—that the Global Fund aims to realize its vision of a partnership between governments, civil society, and patients.

A fourth core feature of the Global Fund's institutional design, now at the global level, is its technical review and resource allocation procedure. A special set of rules govern the interaction between the Fund's Technical Review Panel (TRP), which assesses proposals, and the Fund's Board, which formally approves them for funding or rejects them. The TRP is a panel of experts on health care and international development who receive their mandate from the Fund's board (for details, see the TRP website and terms of reference: The Global Fund to Fight Aids, Tuberculosis and Malaria 2012b, 2012c). It has the authority to judge the technical quality of submitted proposals and to recommend them for funding. In each round, the TRP thus assesses and rates the proposals that have come from local CCMs. Its authority is derived from the expertise of its 26 members, whose experience is rooted in various areas including AIDS, tuberculosis, and malaria as well as "cross-cutting" expertise in management and international development (see, for example, the list of "cross-cutting" experts in the Fund's 2004 annual report: The Global Fund to Fight Aids, Tuberculosis and Malaria 2004a, 57). The TRP reviews the proposals, rates them in four categories, and submits them to the Global Fund's Board for approval.

The authority to make decisions on funding lies with the Fund's Board, which consists of 20 voting members, representing developing countries, donor countries, civil society, the private sector, and patients. However, the board can approve or reject only *categories* of proposals, not *individual* proposals, based on the TRP's rating, which happens on the basis of "global best practices" (see, for example, The Global Fund to Fight Aids, Tuberculosis and Malaria 2004a, 9). The aim of this arrangement is to prevent the board's decisions from being influenced by political considerations concerning single countries and is conceived of as a way to ensure that technical merit is the only criterion for decision making, or as a way of "depoliticizing" the actual funding decisions. The fact that Iran, North Korea, and Myanmar—countries that have been excluded from the international community (and especially the powerful United States, a major contributor to the Fund)—have been able to apply for and receive funding in the past is interpreted by many supporters as proof that the Fund's resource allocation decisions have indeed been successfully "depoliticized."[3] We recognize behind this rule the idea that the new global body will rely on *science only* when distributing resources targeted to delivering health care to the global patient. Donor as well as recipient countries are expected to accept science as a set of global norms, which are conceptualized as neatly separable from the domain of politics.

Technical review is conceptualized as separable from politics not just at the global level, but also at the local level:

> By focusing upon the technical quality of proposals, while leaving the design of programs and priorities to partners reflected by the Country Coordinating Mechanism, the Global Fund also encourages local ownership.
> (The Global Fund to Fight Aids, Tuberculosis and Malaria 2005a)

In the Fund's view, local "ownership," "program design" and "priorities" are not in danger of being compromised in any way by a global technical review procedure. Science is conceived of as transcending nationality, culture and local specificity. Implicit in this idea is also a view of science as uncontroversial and uncontested, an "innocent" form of power. This concept leaves open the exact nature of the relationship between the Fund's "global" expert (the TRP member) and its "local expert" (the CCM-member), on whom the Fund purports to fully rely for the initiation, design and implementation of the programs it finances.[4]

The TRP's evaluation uses political criteria in two major ways: First, the TRP is mandated to approve proposals only if they "reflect genuine, broad participation and ownership of all interested [societal] groups" (The Global Fund to Fight Aids, Tuberculosis and Malaria 2002a, 6); second, it also requires proof of local government's "political commitment" to combating the three diseases covered (The Global Fund to Fight Aids, Tuberculosis and Malaria 2002a, 9). This setup reflects the idea, formulated earlier in the international community, that high-level political commitment is a crucial feature of a successful response to HIV/AIDS (see, for example, Piot 2000). As Chapter 6 will show, it played an important role in China's interaction with the Fund.

The Global Fund and Its Partners

The preceding section focused on the Fund's core, the rules that govern its interaction with the recipients of its money. We now turn to the question of how the Global Fund conceptualizes its relations with other actors in the global health domain. Three categories are listed as the Fund's main partners—the technical agencies (e.g., WHO and UNAIDS), civil society and patients, and the private sector. We see that the Fund assigns roles to them on global as well as local levels. In the process, new identities are created.

Technical Agencies

The Fund relies on a wide variety of bilateral and multilateral agencies including the World Health Organization, the World Bank, UNAIDS, and the UK Department for International Development (DFID) (The Global Fund to Fight Aids, Tuberculosis and Malaria 2002c). At the global level, the Fund relies on UNAIDS, WHO, and others for the definition of "best practice" in public health:

> For technical expertise—both to the Secretariat, to Country Coordinating Mechanisms and potential Principal Recipients—the Global Fund relies on international organizations like the World Health Organization (WHO), UNAIDS, UNDP and the World Bank, which serves as its trustee.
>
> (The Global Fund to Fight Aids Tuberculosis and Malaria 2002c)

Thus, the Fund assigns to the technical agencies that of setting the standards and norms for "best practice" in public health in the global domain. They are seen as the backbone of a global network that transports universal knowledge between global and local levels. The scientific knowledge the Global Fund takes as the basis for its work is conceptualized as situated in these technical agencies, and as freely available to actors at all levels, including the Fund itself. Again, there is an underlying assumption that local as well as global actors draw in substantial ways on the same kind of knowledge.

At the local level, the Global Fund relies on the partnership with local branches of the technical agencies and development organizations for advice to the local applicants, CCM, and principal recipient:

> As a funding mechanism the Fund does not help implement any of the programs it gives grant money to. Instead, the Global Fund relies on international development partners to provide such support to grantees . . . Multilateral development partners and bilateral agencies' complementary support includes:
>
> - technical assistance for monitoring and evaluation,
> - support for capacity building, including human resources as well as product procurement and supply chain management,
> - dissemination of best practices and financial assistance.
>
> (The Global Fund to Fight Aids Tuberculosis and Malaria 2002c)

Thus, the Fund assigns to local chapters of the WHO, UNAIDS, or DFID the role of supporting the work of local actors.

Civil Society Organizations and NGOs

The second group of actors listed as core partners to the Global Fund are civil society organizations and NGOs. They are presented as indispensable partners to a successful public health response to HIV/AIDS:

> Civil Society and NGOs are the foundation upon which effective responses to the three diseases of AIDS, tuberculosis and malaria are being built. Civil Society are the advocates who in many countries stimulated the first recognition and response to HIV and AIDS. It is Civil Society who is the critical implementer of support, prevention and care programmes particularly to the most vulnerable and hard to reach communities.
>
> (The Global Fund to Fight Aids Tuberculosis and Malaria 2002b)

In the Fund's view, the power and skill of civil society and NGOs rest on their ability to initiate action and advocate for people affected by diseases (independent of national governments, if necessary) and to reach individuals that the authorities cannot see or reach out to. The Global Fund goes so far as to state that its own mission cannot be accomplished unless national governments engage civil society and NGOs:

> There has been a significant shift in the way some governments and international institutions recognize and have acted upon the considerable expertise, knowledge and skills that NGOs have. However there remain many Governments who continue to ignore the rich diversity and resources of our communities. Without this recognition and full support from all Governments and international institutions the unique vision of the Global Fund and the integration of nongovernmental organizations (NGOs) in realizing the vision of the Fund, it will always remain a vision rather than a reality.
>
> (The Global Fund to Fight Aids, Tuberculosis and Malaria 2002b)

The Fund postulates that civil society and NGOs should be empowered and supported within the framework of the nation-state. This vision of civil society participation reveals a broad understanding of what counts as public health. The idea that the involvement of patients and communities is a crucial element of a successful national HIV/AIDS response, eloquently formulated by Piot in *Science* at the turn of the millennium (Piot 2000), has been institutionalized.

The Private Sector

The third major group listed as partners of the Global Fund is the private sector. This relationship seems less clearly defined than the relationships with some of the other partners.[5] In the first few years of the Global Fund's existence, financial contributions of the private sector to the Global Fund were modest at less than 1 percent of the total funding (Dyer 2006). At the same time, this seems to be one of the areas where the Fund has been particularly experimental, creating new rules and trying out new models.

A case in point is a program that arguably represents the Fund's most visible partnership with the private sector—its new fundraising campaign, RED. This program, which is done in cooperation with U2 singer Bono, was launched in January 2006, at a time when the Fund was starting to see a drop in government donations (Dyer 2006). Producers of "lifestyle" products like Giorgio Armani, The Gap, and Apple issue a red version of one of their consumer products at elevated prices, a percentage of which is then diverted to the Fund. With the seductive promise to consumers that they will "look good and do good," the campaign seeks to motivate those who are affluent enough to be able to afford these products to contribute in a virtually effortless way to the global support for HIV/AIDS patients all over the world:

With (PRODUCT) RED, consumers can tap into the power of commerce to do something amazing and unprecedented. Our partners have created incredible products that consumers will want and need, which is the beauty of (PRODUCT) RED. We're not asking anyone for a donation or for them to change their behavior. People buy things every day. But now, when they buy (PRODUCT) RED, they will look good and do good—and that's good business.

("Bono and Bobby Shriver Launch (RED)TM in the U.S." 2006)

The campaign's initiators stress that RED, which Bono predicted will raise "hundreds of millions of dollars," is not a charity but a partnership (Dyer 2006, 263). Richard Feachem, former executive director of the Fund, reportedly called it "a business proposition that brings together partners with distinct priorities into a mutually beneficial relationship" (Dyer 2006, 263)—thus, the Fund increases its resources while the companies expand their reach into the existing so-called ethical consumer markets (Dyer 2006, 264).

In that way, the new initiative aims to establish a connection between the lifestyle of the global affluent with their willingness to help the poor. The Fund imagines a "global consumer" to mirror the "global patient" that it aims to serve—an individual with a certain consumption pattern (luxury goods) and a global social conscience (a concern for the victims of the global HIV/AIDS epidemic). This individual makes donations to Fund not on the basis of membership in a nation-state (through government donation based on tax collection), but on the basis of membership to a certain economic class and identity.

Science and Politics in the Global Fund

The Global Fund's institutional design represents a bold attempt to change the dynamics of development aid. Instead of continuing to work through a donor-driven system yielding results that are uncertain at best and unsustainable at worst, the Fund proposes that we can live in a world in which local actors drive effective responses to HIV/AIDS, tuberculosis, and malaria in line with their own specific needs. In co-productionist terms, the Global Fund combines a view of the nature of disease as a multifactorial social, political, and economic issue with a vision of the politics of managing global disease as requiring the participation of multiple state and nonstate actors across local and global scales.

In line with this basic idea, the Global Fund (re)distributes the responsibilities for global public health action among governments, intergovernmental agencies, the private sector, civil society, and patients, thereby creating a new set of interactions between them (a form of global health policy making). Its ability to do so initially comes from its position as a financing mechanism with substantial amounts of resources to distribute. But beyond the sheer power of money, the Global Fund must prove that it works. It must gain the trust of multiple actors and must render itself accountable and legitimate in this domain. As this chapter has sought to illustrate, the Fund's view of the global domain and of its own authority and legitimacy in that domain hinges on an intricate view of the conditional relationships (Shapin and Schaffer 1985) between science and politics.

At the local level, the Fund aims to recruit both the existing power of national structures and the participation of multiple societal actors. Thus, it suggests that the CCM be built on the basis of an existing national disease control structure. However, it also creates concrete mechanisms through which to empower various nongovernmental actors. By requiring that nongovernmental actors be present on the CCM, the Fund aims to give these actors influence on national-level policy making. By allowing for the possibility that the principal recipient of Global Fund resources be an NGO, the Fund aims to institute a way in which resources can flow to the grassroots levels. Finally, by defining conditions (although only under exceptional circumstances) under which NGOs can bypass their governments and apply to the Fund directly, it creates a scenario in which the grassroots levels engage directly with the global entity. While the Fund does not intend to replace governments as the main actors in the provision of health care to the global patient, it does aim to induce governments to draw on their respective civil societies when initiating, designing, and implementing health policy.

At the global level, the Fund conceptualizes science as the basis on which it acts. It does so first by assigning to its TRP the role of judging the quality of local proposals; second, by assigning to the technical agencies the role of setting standards and norms for public health in the global domain; and third, by relying on those same technical agencies as providers of technical advice on design and implementation of health policy to local actors.

The chapter shows that the Global Fund creates rules along two axes—the local/global axis and the science/politics axis. With respect to politics, the Fund adopts an inclusive view on who should be given power to decide health policy. In Walter Scott's terms, the Fund seems to build on the idea that the planning entity (the state or, in this case, the supranational organization itself) cannot hope to be an all-powerful, all-knowing center able to roll out policies that reach the outmost periphery at its own will; rather, it must carefully devise its interventions with help and input from the grassroots levels in order to be successful (Scott 1998).

The Fund is less "experimental" when it comes to conceptualizing science and knowledge. It upholds a traditional view of knowledge according to which scientific knowledge is universal and transcends national and cultural boundaries, whereas local knowledge is seen as particular and place bound. In attempting to define the relationships between the local and the global, science and knowledge, the Fund has created at least three different forms of expertise and expert identity. First, there is the expertise of the "local expert" who is conceptualized as the driver behind initiation, design, and implementation of local health policy. Second, there is the expertise of the technical agencies, such as the WHO and UNAIDS, which are assigned the role of setting standards and norms for health policy at the global level. And third, there is the expertise of the Fund's TRP, which serves as the basis for evaluating and approving (or rejecting) what the "local expert" proposes.

Intimately intertwined with the idea of science as transcending nation and culture is the Fund's view of science as neatly separable from politics, as a set of objective and neutral standards to which local and global players can defer without any difficulty. Implicit in this view is an imagination of science as an innocent form of power, one that can be seen only as "good" and is not likely to be abused, in contrast to the political power that classic bilateral donors wield in the traditional model. This last assumption is most evident in the Fund's idea that funding decisions can be "depoliticized."

This conceptualization of the relationship between science and politics in the global domain is not accidental. The Global Fund's legitimacy and accountability hinge on it. The reliance on science is presented as the way out of the "catch 22" between fostering local ownership (and therefore, curtailing donor control) while at the same time staying accountable to donors (and therefore having to control the quality of local approaches). By claiming that its work is purely based on science, shielded from "political" forms of influence at every level, the Global Fund wants to achieve the global democratic without bowing to the political.

Conclusion

The analysis of the way in which the Fund envisions policy making in the global domain raises many questions about how this model plays out in reality. I will focus on three main questions. The first question is that of whether new ways of framing things really lead to new forms of engagement. The Global Fund wants to create a novel mode of interaction in the global domain. But as Benedict Anderson shows in his study of states and nationhood, the vision and determination of a powerful entity alone does not suffice to create a new kind of community (Anderson 1991). Anderson's state has powerful tools at its command to create the imagined community of a nation, notably print capitalism. However, Anderson argues that it cannot make this vision reality without the "buy in" from the citizens. By the same token, it would seem that the Global Fund needs the buy-in from a variety of actors in the global domain to create, stabilize, and uphold the particular vision of global public health policy that it has developed and inscribed into its design.

If we do assume that the Fund can introduce changes by virtue of its model, then the second question is, what these changes and interactions look like in reality. It is not hard to see that the Global Fund's idea of governance can run counter to Westphalian principles, especially that of noninterference in the internal workings of nation-states. At the most straightforward level, governments of sovereign states may simply not like the idea of engaging civil society in their decision making, or the idea of having a global scientific expert panel judge the validity of their national health policies. Moreover, the assumption that science can serve as a neutral standard to which all can defer is far from unproblematic. For example, what happens if the propositions of the "local expert" differ from what the "TRP expert" regards as a valid national approach to HIV/AIDS? And what if "local experts" disagree about which policies to introduce? Similarly, what happens when the "TRP expert" is not in line with the "WHO expert" on what constitutes best practice in global public health?

Such cases have already happened. In 2004, the Thai Drug User Network, a local Thai NGO, triggered a controversy by submitting a proposal to the Fund for support of a set of HIV/AIDS policies that are substantially different from the country's official line. According to Kerr et al., the proposal asked for US$ 1.4 million for a harm reduction program that included peer-to-peer components, and therefore stood in stark contrast to government policy of the time, which consisted of law enforcement measures targeted to illicit substance use (Kerr et al. 2004, 2005). The NGO submitted a proposal directly to the Fund, arguing that the government's policies with respect to injection drug users were not evidence based. This is an instance of disagreement between two types of local experts as conceived by the Fund.

Similarly, in 2004, *The Lancet* published an article that accused the Global Fund and the WHO of fostering "medical malpractice" in developing countries (Attaran et al. 2004). In this case, the disagreement is between experts at the global level. The standard of care in malaria therapy was in the process of changing, and many Global Fund supported proposals were still based on the use of older drugs, against which resistances existed. The public health experts held the global authority (the Fund and the WHO) accountable for not incorporating changes in best practice immediately into their design. On the other hand, changing a country's antimalarial policy is a complicated and potentially costly process (Williams, Durrheim, and Shretta 2004). Recipient countries who had designed the programs were facing a trade-off between changing policy in the middle of implementation and thereby potentially delaying the delivery of treatment and implementing strategies based on older drugs. The Fund reacted swiftly to this accusation by re-funding and restructuring all of the proposals still relying on older drugs to include the new standard. However, this instance points to a larger unresolved question, that of how a global authority like the Fund conceptualizes uncertainty and risk in the context of changes in scientific knowledge and treatment standards.

The Lancet example is not likely to stay an exception. Rather, the new interconnectedness that the Fund aims to harness for the good of the global patient has many dimensions, and it is hardly possible to foresee all the ways in which the introduction of new rules of engagement will play out in reality. If the Fund works the way it is intended to, it will be a powerful mechanism for standard setting in the global domain. If a new drug was discovered to prevent severe malaria in pregnant women, for example, the Fund could act as a mechanism to enhance the speed with which this drug is adopted at the country level and then accelerate its delivery throughout sub-Saharan Africa. Of course, the evolution of technology is never predictable. What happens, for example, if this hypothetical drug turned out to harm women or their unborn children, either because previously unknown side effects were revealed after its introduction in a particular subpopulation (e.g., African women) or because faulty practices during its manufacture, assembly, and distribution had rendered it toxic?

This prompts the question of how uncertainty and risk are conceptualized in the global domain. In the current controversy over the discovery of tainted batches of Chinese-produced heparin that were linked to U.S. deaths, questions of accountability and responsibility are far from being straightforward or easy to solve (Barboza 2008). However, their basic assignment is clear— the responsibilities lie with the national drug safety institutions in China and the United States. What would happen if the Global Fund was involved in a similar case?

Going beyond the specialized domain of drug safety, the Fund's campaign RED provides a similar example of this problematic. Many of the companies that participate in RED are multinational enterprises that outsource their manufacturing to developing countries. As Katherine Marshall, ethics counselor to the president of the World Bank, put it, "the main ethical pitfall is that these big companies have very far-flung holdings, and there's bound to be questions raised about some aspect of their operations. That puts them to some extent at risk and also puts the cause at risk" (Dyer

2006). Recent allegations that Apple's iPod was manufactured under "slave like" conditions in China ("iPod 'slave' claims investigated" 2006) illustrate the intricacies of this situation. What if the Fund's new "global consumer," in her efforts to support the "global patient" through the acquisition of an (iPOD)RED, at the same time contributed to the exploitation of the Chinese factory worker? No one would argue that the Fund is directly responsible for such a scenario. However, such a situation would pose fundamental questions about the responsibility of global entities in the face of the unintended and unpredictable consequences of their doings.

These and other questions can be examined only through the analysis of the interaction between the Fund and other actors in the global domain. In the following chapter, I first turn to a local actor, China. I examine the emergence of HIV/AIDS in China as background for the analysis, in Chapter 6, of the interaction between the Global Fund and China.

CHAPTER 5

The Local and the Global: HIV/AIDS in China

This chapter sets the background for the analysis of the interaction between the Global Fund and China (Chapter 6). It traces the emergence of China's HIV/AIDS epidemic between 1985, when the first case of HIV was detected, and 2001, when the country started applying to the Fund for money to support its national HIV/AIDS programs. I am looking at this period because it is one of reframing. Over the course of two decades, HIV/AIDS went from being presented as a "foreign problem" to being seen as a general public health issue. For this reframing to happen, HIV/AIDS first needed to be "localized," or understood as a Chinese problem. This required fundamental changes in the way HIV/AIDS, human behavior, and sexuality were imagined, which in turn were intimately intertwined with China's self-image as a socialist society in a period of deep-reaching socioeconomic reform.

The authorities' image of HIV/AIDS in China was initially characterized by a relatively static social model. HIV/AIDS was presented as a foreign disease from which Chinese society was protected by its socialist values. Propagated by China's top health officials and supported by the country's scientific establishment, this initial framing of HIV/AIDS served to establish the view that China's population was at no risk of contracting the disease. Effective HIV/AIDS control was seen to rest on surveillance, border control, education, and law enforcement measures against prostitution and drug use.

Over time, a variety of local actors worked, often in the face of repression, to make a different view of HIV/AIDS available to the central authorities. HIV/AIDS was detected in different segments of the population, including injection drug users, prostitutes, homosexuals, and plasma donors in Central China. Sexually transmitted diseases reemerged in the 1980s after having been virtually nonexistent for two decades. With the increasing visibility of these groups, competing framings of HIV/AIDS emerged. Walls in the planning mentality broke down and gave way to a more dynamic social model, making room for the recognition of local diversity and for the admission of uncertainty. By the end of the 1990s, central-level health officials presented HIV/AIDS as a problem of general public health, intimately intertwined with China's development and in need of immediate attention.

However, the admission that HIV/AIDS could affect anyone in China did not automatically generate agreement on a national strategy. Rather, it prompted a new question: what set of policies was adequate to halt its spread in China? In the continued presence of competing framings of HIV/AIDS, local actors started experimenting with a range of different (often contradictory) approaches at provincial and subprovincial levels. However, China's first Five Year Plan for HIV/AIDS Prevention and Control, which was released at the time of the 2001 UNGASS declaration that laid the ground work for the creation of the Global Fund, still differed in fundamental ways from the "global HIV/AIDS policy paradigm" adopted in that declaration. The following sections look in detail at the evolution of HIV/AIDS in China until that point in time.[1]

"Localizing" HIV/AIDS in China

On the surface, the evolution of China's response to HIV/AIDS is not unlike that of many other countries, following a pattern that leads from denial to acceptance that Jonathan Mann described in the mid-1980s (Mann 1987a). Transferring psychological thinking about the individual to governments and populations, Mann observed that "a three-part evolution in perspective regarding AIDS can be observed at the personal, national and international levels. The initial response to AIDS usually involves denial . . . Then, as the number of AIDS cases increases rapidly and estimates of the number of persons already infected with HIV in the population are publicized, the HIV problem commands further attention. Finally, once the virus' potential to involve major segments of the population, including those who may have previously considered themselves without risk, is recognized, the epidemic nature and urgency of the HIV situation generate political commitment and a willingness to act."

While this pattern can certainly be used to describe the evolution of China's public representation of HIV/AIDS, there are also some very unique characteristics to it that are connected to China's political system, culture, and the tremendous socioeconomic changes the country has been going through since the 1980s. UNAIDS's 2002 assessment of the Chinese HIV/AIDS epidemic shows that the disease is best understood as several simultaneous epidemics (see United Nations Joint Programme on AIDS (UNAIDS) 2002). Thus, a mainly injection-drug use-driven epidemic originated in the border areas of southern provinces of Yunnan and Sichuan and spread throughout the country during the 1980s via channels such as prostitution along truck routes; in parallel, a separate epidemic developed among poor peasants in Henan and six other Central Chinese provinces throughout the 1990s, caused by unsafe blood donation practices; finally, a sexual epidemic has been spreading in the general population. By 2004, China was officially reporting 1 million HIV/AIDS cases (Country Coordinating Mechanism in China 2005). But this low prevalence of less than 1 percent disguised high infection rates in certain localizations, such as the Central Chinese provinces (Kaufman, Kleinman, and Saich 2006), and it has been suggested that the actual number was substantially higher (United Nations Joint Programme on AIDS (UNAIDS) 2002; Kaufman and Jing 2002). But in 2005, the official numbers were down revised to 650,000 (see Wu et al. 2007).

As Saich et al. have argued, the unique epidemiological pattern of the Chinese HIV/AIDS epidemic is intimately intertwined with the tremendous political, economic, and social changes that began in the 1980–1990s, when the country started transforming its economy from a centrally planned, Soviet-style system to a more market driven one (see Saich 2006). First, notwithstanding substantial gains in the general standard of living, the economic reforms of the 1980s and 1990s led to the emergence of disadvantaged groups, whose economic situation has made them more vulnerable to HIV/AIDS—these groups include a growing number of rural poor, a population of about 200 million internally migrating workers, and a new class of urban poor (see Saich 2006). Second, the reforms also created strains for public finance that undermined the public health system and created incentives that led officials to favor the emphasis on economic targets over the protection of health and well-being of citizens. This pressure played an important role in the spread of HIV/AIDS through blood and blood products in Central China (Saich 2006, 27; see also Zhang 2005).

This chapter follows the change in representation of HIV/AIDS in China and the responses that were formulated in the context of the changing representations. Chinese authorities published in striking detail not only the numbers of infected individuals but also their national origin, the route of transmission, the geographic location where the infection had taken place, and the nationality of the source of the infection. At each point in time, a "snapshot" of the epidemic was thus made public. In Foucauldian terms, this snapshot reflected where the state had directed its gaze (Foucault 1979), what it had *looked for,* and where it was therefore finding HIV/AIDS.

By virtue of its tendency to affect those who are economically or socially vulnerable, HIV/AIDS brought to the fore many problems the Chinese government wished it did not have, like injection drug use and prostitution. It also made visible behaviors that were regarded as immoral and undesirable, such as changes in sexual norms among Chinese men and women, including an increasingly open display of homosexual identity. Over time, different populations became visible to the public eye. Some had been there before, like homosexual men, injection drug users, or prostitutes and their clients. But other populations were new, like former plasma donors and their children in the so-called AIDS villages in Central China. The us/other boundary between those affected and those not affected (described in Chapter 2) was first presented as a stark boundary congruent with different categories, including national identity, morality, sexual preference, and gender. Over time, it kept moving as the imagined map of the Chinese AIDS epidemic changed from an essentially blank space to one that showed every Chinese province and every societal group before it finally came to be substituted by a more inclusive "we."

Foreigners

On June 6, 1985, the first case of HIV/AIDS was reported in the Chinese press. According to the Chinese Ministry of Health, an Argentinean tourist who had been diagnosed to be HIV positive in the United States died of AIDS-related respiratory failure at Peking Union College Hospital ("China says Argentine died of AIDS" 1985). For many years to come, China's public health and scientific establishment presented HIV/AIDS as a foreigner's disease. Zeng Yi, vice president of the Chinese Academy of Preventive Medical Sciences and an eminent national infectious disease specialist, said that AIDS had "no sources" for the spread of HIV/AIDS ("Scientist says China has no AIDS 'sources'" 1988). HIV/AIDS, he stated, was "a foreign threat" that could enter the country only "from foreigners" (Schweisberg 1988) and that it had entered China through infected blood products and through casual sex with the growing number of foreign nationals now present in the country ("China steps up anti-AIDS measures" 1988).

This initial representation of HIV/AIDS as a foreign disease was based on the idea that it was rooted in values and behaviors common in the Western political system, but not in China. In 1987, an article in the Beijing Review spoke of the "decadent" American society in which "rampant disastrous drug taking, alcoholism, robbery, homicide, suicide, divorce, prostitution, homosexuality, syphilis, AIDS, and other social ills . . . come from their ideology" (Anderson 1987). Similarly, Health Minister Chen Minzhang argued that in theory, HIV/AIDS could spread in China via the three routes of imported blood products, contaminated injection equipment, and sexual intercourse between Chinese women and foreign men; he suggested, however, that an epidemic in the general population was unlikely because its major routes of transmission, gay sex and sex with multiple partners, were not common behaviors in Chinese society ("Aids can be checked in China—experts" 1987). The us/other boundary was constructed as being identical with the boundary between China and the outside world.

This representation of HIV/AIDS suggested that China's general public was not in danger. It also suggested that focusing on China's geographic and regulatory borders was the best strategy to protect China from AIDS. Consequently, China's first strategy for tackling HIV/AIDS rested on four pillars: surveillance, border control, education, and measures against prostitution. The authorities set up a number of national-level institutions in order to coordinate surveillance measures. In 1986 and 1987, a National AIDS Committee and a National Programme for AIDS Prevention and Control were set up (Zhang 2004). In 1988, a new National Center for the Prevention and Treatment of Sexually Transmitted Diseases was added in Nanjing, which ran 16 surveillance stations in rural areas and eight in major cities ("China acts up to crackdown on sexually transmitted diseases" 1988). To support their work, the Ministry of Health announced, in 1989, that a new law now empowered Chinese officials to require any citizen to undergo an HIV test: "if local authorities want someone tested, he must be tested. He has no right to refuse . . . If any Chinese is found to be an AIDS sufferer, he will be quarantined and will not be allowed to continue working or going to school" (Wilhelm 1989). The quote clearly illustrates the underlying law enforcement mind set (the state assumes the right to test individual citizens), which draws an *us/other boundary* to separate the patient from the community. These measures formed the basis for HIV/AIDS surveillance throughout the 1980s and 1990s. The authorities initially tested specific groups, mainly foreigners and Chinese individuals who were known to have been outside of China, like sailors (see, for example, "China makes efforts to prevent aids" 1987), and later patients with sexually transmitted diseases (STDs), blood donors, gay individuals, as well as prostitutes and their clients ("Risk Groups to be Eyed for AIDS" 1990).

The second pillar of early Chinese HIV/AIDS policy was stricter border control for both individuals and goods. By September 1987, China had adopted several regulations and measures. These included the prohibition for HIV-infected individuals to enter China, a ban on any introduction into China of foreign blood or blood products and "second-hand clothing," the prohibition of "illegal sexual contacts with foreigners," and a requirement for all medical institutions that accept foreigners to sterilize their equipment and "use syringes only once" ("China makes efforts to prevent AIDS" 1987).

Public education efforts, the third pillar at the time, matched the trend. While officials and the press frequently reported on HIV/AIDS, there was no suggestion that its presence in the country carried lessons of any relevance to the everyday life of the average Chinese citizen unless he or she interacted with foreigners. For example, a widely seen movie entitled "the AIDS Patients" narrated the story of three young Chinese women infected with HIV/AIDS by their foreign teacher ("'Controversial' AIDS Film Fills Cinemas" 1989).

The fourth pillar of China's early response to HIV/AIDS consisted of law enforcement measures against prostitution. In 1987, the Ministry of Health announced that the enforcement of Article 30 of the Regulations on Public Order to Prevent AIDS in China, an article that forbids casual sex and prostitution, was a crucial part of China's efforts against HIV/AIDS (Macartney 1987). According to one source, more than 580,000 sex workers were detained in China between 1981 and 1991 (Cohen et al. 2000, 144). This approach makes sense in light of China's history. China had staggering rates of STDs in the 1940s, with syphilis rates of around 5 percent in cities, 2–3 percent in rural areas, and as high as 10 percent among the adult population in some minority communities (see Cohen et al. 1996, S224). Under Mao Zedong, the Communist Party framed prostitution and STDs as a direct consequence of China's contact with the West and with Western imperialism (see Cohen et al. 1996, 143; also Cohen et al. 2000). The newly instituted Communist regime virtually eliminated STDs through a program that was based on testing, antibiotic therapy, and radical measures against prostitution in the context of increasing seclusion of the country from the outside world (see Cohen et al. 1996, 2000).

International health experts certainly did not share the Chinese authorities' interpretation of HIV/AIDS as a Western scourge, but they did agree that a heterosexual HIV/AIDS epidemic in China was preventable. As part of a 1988 announcement on planned cooperation with the Chinese government, WHO Chairman on AIDS programs Jonathan Mann said, "up to now we have not seen AIDS spread in China, so it is not too late for China to prevent it" ("WHO and China join hands in fight against AIDS" 1988). China was seen as being in a relatively good position to control HIV/AIDS, due to its comparatively strong infrastructure and high levels of governmental control (see, for example, Kaufman and Jing 2002). The fact that China was regarded as having successfully eradicated STDs in its past (see, for example, Cohen et al. 1996, 2000) arguably also played a role in these assessments.

Until 1990, this representation of HIV/AIDS as a foreigner's problem remained largely unchallenged, and the majority of new cases were presented as part of it.[2] In December 1989, the official number of cases was 32; according to the Ministry of Health, six of these were Chinese individuals, of which four had contracted HIV through foreign blood products, one had been infected during a visit to Africa, and one "reportedly had engaged in homosexual activities" ("VD cases multiply in China" 1989; "Public warned to be on guard against AIDS" 1989). This latter case appears to have been China's first publicly documented "indigenous" case of sexually transmitted HIV/AIDS. Vice Director of the Department of Epidemic Prevention in the Ministry of Public Health Cao Qing explained to the press that the man "was detained for committing homosexual acts, a crime in China" ("China Discovers First AIDS Virus Carrier" 1989).

Perpetrators

In February 1990, the official number of HIV/AIDS cases suddenly rose from 32 to 194. Dai Zhicheng, the head of the Epidemic Prevention Department at the Ministry of Health, said that 146 HIV cases had been detected among local injection drug users in Yunnan province ("China reports 194 infected by AIDS virus" 1990). Public health authorities had only recently started to look for HIV in Southern China's growing population of injection drug users.[3] In June 1990, *China Daily* reported that a total of 91 additional cases had been detected near the Golden Triangle ("Ninety-one more drug addicts found infected with AIDS" 1990). Similar epidemics later developed in nine other provinces, with HIV rates of up to 70 percent detected in injection drug users (see Kaufman and Jing 2002).

With this information having surfaced, the framing of HIV/AIDS changed slightly. Chinese health experts started presenting HIV/AIDS as a penalty for unwanted behavior and its prevention as a matter of encouraging "healthy" behavior. At a Sino-U.S. meeting on HIV/AIDS, which took place in Beijing in November 1990, convening experts from the domains of medicine, law, education, and social and religious studies, Wang Xiaodao, a professor at Beijing Medical University and an expert on the Chinese National Sexual Science Committee, referred to AIDS as a form of punishment by nature ("Sino-American AIDS symposium opens in Beijing" 1990; "Healthy behavior key to aids eradication" 1990). At the same meeting, a professor at the National Health Education Institute of China, Zhu Qi, argued it was impossible to control HIV/AIDS with medicines and condoms—"only through healthy lifestyle can humanity survive the AIDS epidemic" ("Healthy behavior key to aids eradication" 1990). This interpretation of HIV/AIDS as "social" (not biomedical) served to uphold an imagined boundary between moral and immoral, legal and illegal, behavior.

Again, it is instructive to compare this representation with previous representations of the connections between ideology, sexuality, and STDs in China's history. As others have previously described, the Communist Party, building on Confucian and Taoist ideas, placed sexuality firmly in the context of reproduction and presented sexual activity for the sake of individual pleasure as detrimental to both the health of the individual and the fabric of society (see, for example, Renaud, Byers, and Pan 1997; Parish et al. 2007). During the cultural revolution, a "non-sexuality culture" had emerged in which the mere act of thinking of sexuality was deemed harmful and undesirable (see Parish and Pan 2006, 207).

Socialist values were now no longer presented as a shield that would protect China against the entry of HIV/AIDS from the outside world, but as a set of values that gave China comparative advantage over the West in stemming an HIV/AIDS epidemic. In November 1990, China Central Television (CCTV) broadcasted an emission during which Chen Minzhang, the minister of health, explained that the superiority of the Chinese socialist system made HIV/AIDS controllable in China ("Health Officials on Measures to Control Spread of AIDS" 1990). The geographic us/them boundary was mapped onto a moral one: that between the Chinese general population and perceived perpetrators who violated legal and societal norms—injection drug users, prostitutes, and homosexuals. The possibility of a heterosexual HIV/AIDS epidemic in China was still considered unlikely. When *Xinhua News* reported on China's first two female victims of HIV/AIDS, it clearly stated that the women had been infected as a consequence of their husbands' injection drug use behavior ("Two HIV cases detected in Yunnan" 1990). In the previously mentioned TV emission, the China CDC's Dai Zhicheng said:

> Like other venereal diseases, AIDS is closely related to social activities. In Western countries, AIDS is a disease that is very hard to control. In our country, because of the superiority of our socialist system, we can take comprehensive measures to control it. For example, an anti-pornography drive is being developed throughout the entire society. I believe that this is an effective measure for eliminating AIDS and other venereal diseases. It is imperative to firmly ban such unhealthy or criminal acts as prostitution, visiting prostitutes and using drugs. Also, it is necessary to enact legislation to ban them. This is the radical way to eliminate the soil for growing AIDS.
>
> ("Health Officials on Measures to Control Spread of AIDS" 1990)

Dai's "pornography drive" refers to a nationwide campaign named "sweeping away the yellow subjects," which had been launched at the end of 1989 and which banned all forms of written, audio, or visual expression of any kind of sexual behavior (Pan 1993). The quote renders visible the way in which the government imagined the relation between education and individual behavior. Preventing individuals from viewing pornographic materials is seen as an effective means of preventing them from engaging in unwanted sexual behavior. Thus, one of the rationales behind the pornography campaign was the argument that viewing "yellow" (that is, pornographic) subjects could turn certain individuals into sex offenders (Pan 1993). This approach is in line with an "education as prevention" strategy, which rests on the belief that transporting uniform (socialist) sexual knowledge across the masses directly affects and regulates the sexual behavior of individuals (see, for example, Gil 1994, 14). It also betrays the top-down planning mentality of a state that believes it can effectively see and control the behavior of its population from the center and an image of Chinese society as unchanged with respect to earlier periods in its history.

Meanwhile, doubting voices had started to appear outside and inside the country. The World Health Organization's (WHO) view started to diverge from the government's official representation of HIV/AIDS in China, partly informed by the fact that its view of HIV/AIDS in *Asia* had shifted. In 1992, *The New York Times* printed a special report entitled "Edge of the Chasm— AIDS Comes to Asia," which stated that the health agency was concerned that in some parts of Asia, HIV could be rising at a speed comparable to that seen in sub-Saharan Africa at the outset of the epidemic (Shenon 1992). In the article, Michael Merson, then director of WHO's Global Program on AIDS, was quoted as saying, "in Asia, millions of people will get AIDS and millions of people will die" and the epidemic could deliver a severe blow to governments, health infrastructure, and the labor force across the region.

As Asia's most populous and powerful nation, China became a focus of attention. In 1993, the WHO stated that an estimated 15,000 individuals were infected in China, whereas the China Ministry of Health spoke of only 5,000 ("Drug abuse, prostitutes, migration cause AIDS peril in China" 1993). International health experts increasingly started pointing to populations beyond China's injection drug users. UN representative Bernard Kean warned that time was running out, arguing that China's growing prostitution and increasingly affluent and expanding mobile population could become vulnerable to HIV ("Time running out for China to fight AIDS" 1992).

At the same time, local health experts also modified their view of HIV/AIDS. Chinese social scientists were becoming aware of the potential interconnections between the spread of HIV/AIDS and the social and economic changes that were taking place in China at the time. In December 1992, *Xinhua News* published a news release informing its readers that researchers at the Economic Institute of the Chinese Academy of Social Sciences recommended that research be done to better understand the cost of the epidemic's spread, as well as its effects on "labor markets, investment practices... economic growth... rural labor flow to cities, and the relationship between infection and high-labor-flow jobs" ("Chinese economists join AIDS research" 1992). Their effort can be seen as an attempt to induce the state to look for HIV/AIDS in populations where it had not looked before.

These opinions became visible to the public through the press. In November 1993, *Xinhua News Agency* reported that an official from the Research Office of the State Council, who remained anonymous, had urged for more focus on AIDS prevention; he warned that curbing the disease was a "strategic issue in China's modernization" and that the failure to address it in time could result in a "disaster for the Chinese nation and a threat to the current reform and opening drive" ("Failure to curb AIDS can sabotage socialist construction—official" 1993).

During the early 1990s, a lack of clear guidance from the central government created a gray zone in which proactive officials were able to maneuver with considerable degree of freedom. For example, Wan Yanhai, an employee of the Ministry of Health's National Health Education Institute, and later to become one of the country's most prominent HIV/AIDS activists, led the design of a national plan to actively engage homosexual men in HIV/AIDS prevention conducted by his agency ("China's homosexuals urged to come out of closet, help with AIDS education" 1993). The plan targeted Beijing, Shanghai, and Guangdong provinces and previewed the institution of counseling centers, telephone hotlines, research, and free condom distribution ("China's homosexuals urged to come out of closet, help with AIDS education" 1993). As Wan later described in an interview with *Seed Magazine* (Rosenberg 2002), Wan and his colleagues worked closely with public security authorities to gain access to homosexuals, injection drug users, and prostitutes, even bringing together gay rights activists (who worked covertly in Beijing) and the police in efforts to establish peer education programs in the gay community. In the interview, Wan also recalls that participating public security officials had told him: "We're in a time of reforming everything, so you can try."

However, this situation did not last long. Difficulties arose from the perception that public health officials were moving into the human rights domain. In August 1993, Chen Bingzhong, the director of the National Health Education Institute and Wan's employer, lost his job after accusations that he had made HIV/AIDS prevention a pretext for furthering the rights of homosexuals (Chandra 1993; Crothall 1993). The measure received support from a number of Chinese as well as Western social scientists and political analysts, who held that Wan and Chen were advertising measures that had not worked in the West and that "making AIDS a political and civil rights issue, as gay rights groups have done in the West, has prevented the authorities from taking effective action to curb the epidemic" (Crothall 1993).

Victims

While these controversies over the sexual transmission of HIV/AIDS in China were ongoing, a devastating epidemic quietly unfolded among plasma donors in Central China throughout the first half of the 1990s. Between 1992 and 1996, thousands of poor farmers contracted HIV in the context of a blood and plasma product industry that formed part of the provinces' efforts to spur economic development (Zhang 2005). Until today, relatively little is known about this epidemic as access to the areas and to information has been restricted. One of the few first-hand accounts is the testimony of Zhang Ke, an infectious diseases physician at Beijing You'an Hospital (Zhang 2005). According to his own account, Zhang became aware of the problem in 1999, after a group of villagers from Henan contacted him in Beijing, requesting to be tested for HIV. Over the course of five years, he visited more than 100 villages in Henan province on multiple occasions despite repeated attempts by local authorities to intimidate him—interacting with patients, their families, and local officials; training local doctors; and documenting the epidemic. He has described his work in a report entitled "Report on AIDS in Henan after a Five-Year Investigation" (Zhang 2005), which I draw on in the following section.

Henan province lies in the center of China. As described earlier, the economic development targets that had been set by the central government in the 1990s had created pressure for the authorities of the region: as these poor areas were not being able to attract foreign investment in the way that some of the booming cities and provinces on China's coast were able to do, their local governments needed to devise other strategies to progress in terms of their economic development (Saich 2006). Partially as a way out of this problem, Henan and several other provinces initiated what Zhang terms a *plasma economy:* a business sector that collected and sold human blood and its derivatives for use in the pharmaceuticals sector—this included whole blood for classic blood transfusions, as well as blood plasma and biological substances commonly derived from plasma, such as *factor VIII* for the treatment of hemophilia (Zhang 2005).

Zhang's account suggests that the Henan health authorities played an active role in shaping and implementing this strategy. In June 1992, a report entitled "Act Fast to Speed Up Health Reforms and to Contribute to the Promotion of Our Province to a Higher Step Economically," authored by the Henan Health Department and discussed in a meeting of senior leaders, presented the case for the new economic branch, explaining how it would "introduce foreign capital, technology, personnel and management experience" and "encourage foreign investment from Hong Kong, Macao and Taiwan" (Zhang 2005, 5). On the basis of this thinking, local health authorities actively took part in jump-starting the *plasma economy*. Zhang recounts:

> In the early 1990, with the whole country advocating "becoming rich rapidly" . . . blood centres operated by the health sector went to the remote and poor central areas, where cheap and clean blood was ideal for blood collection. To mobilize the farmers to donate their blood, the local government actively set up blood centres, and gave strong support to the building up of the blood centres. Some local government officials went to cut the ribbon at an opening ceremony in person, to encourage the setting-up of blood centres.
>
> (Zhang 2005, 5)

The quote illustrates how local health authorities were lending government credibility to the new blood centers. However, they also provided credibility on the blood donor side. Thus, in order to be able to donate blood, individuals had to obtain health certificates from the provincial authorities, and some farmers had as many as 10 certificates for different localities within the province (Zhang 2005, 10). This conferred an official touch on the entire *plasma economy* and inspired confidence in the system.

Zhang's testimony shows that the local authorities did not just provide credibility to the new businesses, but also actively fostered them and invested resources in their creation. Indeed, his account suggests that the boundaries between public policy and private sector activity quickly became blurred. In December 1992, the disease control authorities of Zhukou Prefecture and the Zhukou *Provincial Biological Products Centre*, a local enterprise, cooperated in the initiation of a "white cell production line"—with 7 billion CNY of capital accumulated (Zhang 2005, 6), suggesting that public and private interests became very closely intertwined in the context of this venture. And the following account by the *Henan Health Paper*, transmitted by Zhang, of a signing ceremony for the first subcontracted blood station in Henan province illustrates the strong public endorsement by the authorities that the new economic branch of the province enjoyed:

> In the ceremony, Mr. Xu, Deputy Director of the Department of Health, signed the contract, together with Mr. Zhang, person in charge of the blood centre. This paved the way for developing blood products in our province, and to transform the technology, equipment advantage and potential for commercial products. In the contracted period (one year), the blood centre will produce 1000 kg of albumin and 250 kg of globulin worth 20 million Yuan. This exceeded the all-time record high by two times.
>
> (Zhang 2005, 5)

Besides conferring capital and credibility, the local authorities also helped make the new practice acceptable in the rural population. It appears that the health authorities' initial efforts to channel the blood product activity under their own umbrella and auspices were soon lost in a growing tide of uncontrolled activity, as new blood centers rapidly opened unofficially across the province. The following account by Zhang shows how a village-level party official took the initiative to set up a blood business in his own community and mobilized everyone, including his own family, to become part of the deadly cycle:

> Influenced by the blood centres opened by the government, together with the fact that the management was not very strict, numerous underground blood centres emerged, like bamboo shoots emerging after rain . . . They often opened these blood centres in villagers' homes or fields, and collected blood around the clock. Li Kelin, the party secretary of Xiaoli village of Henan at that time, invited private blood heads[4] on his own initiative and set up a blood centre in his home to help his villagers to get rich and to make it more convenient for the villagers to sell their blood. The blood centre was working 24 hours. His action did not bring wealth to the villagers, but brought HIV to more than 100 people in the village, including himself and his six brothers. In Weishi County, at that time, there were only three blood centres operated by the health sector, but there were 20–30 privately run underground blood centres.
>
> (Zhang 2005, 6)

The villagers happily responded to the new opportunity to increase their low incomes. Zhang describes how individuals of all ages joined a veritable movement of "blood for wealth," how the sight of people lining up for blood donation became common in the villages, and how the elderly would dye their hair to circumvent restrictions on age that kept them from being admitted as donors (Zhang 2005, 6). Unfortunately, the private enterprises were badly equipped and negligent with respect to the safety of their practices. A local official, quoted in *The New York Times*, vividly described an eerie contrast between the enthusiasm that prevailed among villagers to become plasma donors and the lack of professionalism and human dignity of the settings in which the plasma donations were performed:

> Villagers became crazy about selling blood because they are so poor and life is so hard. Many had built their houses by selling blood. Some will even bribe traffickers to be able to sell more than once a day. Once we saw hundreds of people lined up there at the entrance of our village. I thought it must be a vegetable market or a movie. It turned out to be blood selling! I felt so terrified because there is no sterilized equipment at all. Villagers just tell the traffickers their blood type and then lie down on the ground to offer blood.
>
> (Rosenthal 2000b)

The lack of sterilized equipment and the lack of systematic testing alone would arguably not have been enough to explain a rapid spread of HIV in the population. Zhang identifies two practices that, combined together, can explain rapid transmission (Zhang 2005, 8). First, the new enterprises pooled the blood cells of large numbers of donors and re-injected them into donating individuals afterward. As Zhang explains, this was done to simplify procedures and to increase the throughput of the equipment for plasma donations—those who signed up to donate plasma only, a practice that was particularly popular because it could be repeated more frequently than whole blood donation, were thus injected with blood cells of their own blood group after they had donated whole blood. This way the businesses would "net out" with a plasma donation only, and the donor could come back in short intervals. However, given the businesses did not test the collected blood for HIV or other infections, this practice meant that once a single HIV-positive individual became part of this donation pool, the transmission rate was greatly amplified, and everyone who received a re-injection of blood cells from that pool was immediately infected. The second factor that Zhang identified as a major contributor to rapid transmission of the virus throughout the province was the fact that donors also traveled in groups to the different localities, in order to increase their incomes and to help businesses maintain a steady output of product; this highly increased the chances that HIV and other infections were spread to different centers and entered into the various donation pools. Taken together, these practices contributed to a sharp rise in HIV/AIDS and other infections, in the province.

Before 1994, no case of HIV was detected, arguably because no one looked for it. In principle, the danger of the spread of infectious diseases through this route was known to the local health authorities. Surveillance by local branches of the national CDC revealed increasing rates of malaria and syphilis in Henan early into the years of the *plasma economy* (Zhang 2005, 9). However, the decision to test blood donors for HIV and Hepatitis C was not made until August 1993 (Zhang 2005, 9). In 1994, Wang Shuping, a health official at the CDC in the Zhukou Prefecture, found HIV among local plasma donors. According to Zhang's testimony, Wang reported this finding to the local authorities, who dismissed it. She then sent the samples to Zeng Yi at the Chinese Academy of Sciences in Beijing. From there, the news arrived at the central health authorities, who issued the direction that Henan should ban all paid blood donations immediately and close the blood centers (Zhang 2005).

The local authorities removed Wang from her post (she was later hired by Zeng Yi to work in Beijing). Without making mention of her findings, the provincial health department then made an emergency announcement that all plasma-only collection be stopped, except those centers producing blood supply for immediate clinical use (Zhang 2005, 18). But according to Zhang, these measures had no real consequences. Given the continued existence of government blood donation centers and the lack of concrete measures to accompany the regulation, the activity continued unchanged until about 1996 (Zhang 2005).

According to Zhang's estimates, 300,000 farmers contracted the virus in Henan alone.[5] The majority of them were infected *after* Wang's initial discovery, during the period of 1994–1995, with 1995 being the peak of infections (Zhang 2005, 10). Zhang's report makes clear that the health authorities at central as well as local levels were aware of the situation throughout the second half of the 1990s, but chose to repress the information. Thus, Zhang received a letter from the Ministry of Health ordering him to stop visiting Henan as his visits were hindering local efforts to prevent HIV/AIDS.[6]

Despite official warnings and threatening phone calls to his home, Zhang continued his work. Over the period 1999–2003, he visited over 100 villages in Central China, providing medical help and collecting evidence. Zhang recalls urging provincial officials to expose the catastrophe in order to get assistance from Beijing and from outside the country. However, fear of economic repercussions was great. One official said: "You can never do that [expose the epidemic]. Once this is disclosed, nobody will invest here, and we will lose out on economic development." Some officials also placed little value on the lives of affected farmers. One official told Zhang: "Dr. Zhang, no problem, after two years, when they are all dead, there will be no problem." The cynical statement of this particular official, he suggests, reflected a general attitude among provincial officials to prioritize their career prospects, which were linked to fulfillment of central-level targets, over the rights and well-being of the population they governed:

> The words of the official illustrated the thinking of the majority of the local officials, because their jobs and future promotions are linked with economic development targets. As for the fact that AIDS was killing people, or how many people it was killing, that did not matter to him because it was not linked with his achievements or his post, and would not be linked to his promotion. Of course, there are not a few officials who admitted that if the situation were exposed, they might be held responsible. This is another reason why local governments will continue to avoid working on AIDS in the future.
>
> (Zhang 2005, 19)

There were other individuals besides Zhang who tried to bring the news of the epidemic outside of Henan. In particular, Dr. Gao Yaojie, a retired gynecologist who had seen the first case of a Henan woman dying of AIDS in 1996, started to provide support to patients to the extent her means allowed (Rosenthal 2000b). She also started publishing an HIV/AIDS newsletter on the Internet, in cooperation with Wan Yanhai, who had by then started an NGO named "Aids Action Project" in Beijing (Rosenberg 2002). However, Henan officials threatened Gao to stop her activities, fearing that they would harm the province's business and economic development (Rosenthal 2000a, 2000b). Dr. Gao later received an award for her work from the Vital Voices Global Partnership in New York but was denied permission to leave the country to receive it (Yardley 2007). The Chinese authorities were not willing to make details of the local plasma donation-related epidemics visible to the outside.

The General Population

The news of the Henan plasma donors did not really surface to the press and public until the year 2000. But meanwhile, another development pointed to the possibility of HIV/AIDS affecting the general population. In February 1994, the *Beijing Daily* reported an "appalling rise in sexually transmitted diseases" in the country, which was transported in the international press (see "Venereal disease in China more than doubling every two years" 1994). As a study of the Institute of Dermatology of the Chinese Academy of Medical Sciences later showed, STD rates rose rapidly in the period between 1989 and 1998, after having been virtually nonexistent in the 1960s and 1970s (Chen et al. 2000).

Scholars link the rise in STDs to changes in societal values and norms that happened in the context of China's socioeconomic transition. For example, Parish and Pan argue that after the one-child policy had had the unforeseen side effect of separating sex and reproduction in people's minds, a "sexual revolution" happened in China in the mid-1980s as a consequence of increasing contact with culture and media from the outside (Parish and Pan 2006, 207).

A second factor posited as an explanation for rising STD rates in China was prostitution (Cohen et al. 2000; Huang et al. 2004; Parish and Pan 2006; Parish et al. 2007). Some of the societal groups whose emergence is closely intertwined with China's economic reforms are seen as particularly prone to using their services. These include a "surplus" of millions of young, poor, and unmarried men who make up a big part of the country's internal migrating population (Tucker et al. 2005); truck drivers traversing routes between Southern Chinese provinces and other regions of China (visiting brothels or trafficking drugs on their way) (Gil 1994); and (mentioned only more recently) relatively affluent government officials and urban men and their changing sexual behaviors (Kaufman and Jing 2002; Parish and Pan 2006).

By the mid-1990s, amidst competing framings of HIV/AIDS, we increasingly see a connection being made between HIV/AIDS, STDs, and heterosexual sex. In March 1994, the WHO used the news of rising STD rates to officially warn China that it could be facing a serious HIV/AIDS epidemic ("WHO warns China it faces AIDS epidemic." 1994). In July of the same year, the Ministry of Health said China needs to abandon its "prudish attitude towards sex education" to prevent HIV/AIDS from rising ("China's AIDS experts call for education" 1994). According to United Press International, Guangdong local media reported that "experts are very worried because the great majority of people have no feeling of crisis and hold that the disease is a foreigner's illness" (Holland 1994).

Congruent with this shift in the representation of HIV/AIDS, the central government introduced a number of high-level measures signaling that HIV/AIDS and STDs were a matter of concern to the government. In 1995, the Ministry of Health published "Suggestions for Enhancing the Prevention and Control of HIV/AIDS," which were, for the first time, authorized by the State Council (China Ministry of Health & UN Theme Group on HIV/AIDS in China 2003, 19). In 1996, the State Council Coordination Mechanism on AIDS/STD was established on the basis of 34 ministries and commissions (China Ministry of Health & UN Theme Group on HIV/AIDS in China 2003, 23), which later became the basis for the establishment of the China Country Coordinating Mechanism (Country Coordinating Mechanism in China 2003). In 1997, the Chinese Ministry of Health cooperated with the UN Theme Group on HIV/AIDS in China to produce a report in preparation of a donor meeting on HIV/AIDS in China, which was to take place in Beijing in 1998 (China Ministry of Health & UN Theme Group on HIV/AIDS in China 1997). There was also a slight increase in financial resources for HIV/AIDS prevention and control, from CNY 5 Million to CNY 15 Million.[7]

Central Directives, Local Perspectives

By the end of 1996, public health officials had turned around. Minister of Health Chen Minzhang was quoted in several newspapers as saying:

A general unawareness of HIV/AIDS, drug abuse, prostitution, illegal blood supply and the drastic increase of sexually transmitted disease cases may also contribute to the HIV/AIDS epidemic . . . it could be the last chance. We have no time to waste.

("Officials say China has no time to waste to control AIDS" 1996)

This was a far cry from Chen's earlier interpretation of HIV/AIDS as a foreigner's illness requiring a "pornography drive" throughout the population. China's rhetoric toward the outside changed. When China's Vice Health Minister Yin Daikui visited the 12th AIDS Conference in Geneva with the news that of 10 million Chinese tested for HIV, 9,970 were positive, he also mentioned that the proportion of sexual transmission of HIV was rising annually ("China aims to keep HIV infections below 1.5 million by 2010" 1998).

The government's focus on targets and end points was unchanged. Yin stated that the target was to keep the HIV prevalence among adults in China below 0.2 percent, in the best case below 1.5 million in 2010, and announced a new plan with medium-term objectives of halting the transmission of HIV/AIDS via blood products and via injection drug use and reducing the rate of STDs to fewer than 15 percent ("China aims to keep HIV infections below 1.5 million by 2010" 1998). As Vice Health Minister Yin Daikui reported to the 12th AIDS Conference in Geneva, the Chinese government had invested US$ 5.6 million on HIV/AIDS prevention and control since 1987 ("China spends nearly 5.6 million U.S. dollars on HIV/AIDS prevention" 1998).

In November 1998, the State Council issued a "Long- and Medium Term Plan for HIV/AIDS Prevention and Control (1998–2010)" (State Council of China 1998), which required that government at all levels make HIV/AIDS prevention and control an integral part of their social and economic development policy (State Council of China 1998; United Nations Joint Programme on AIDS (UNAIDS) 2002, 32).[8] These measures were still mainly based on surveillance and education. However, for the first time, there was an explicit, central-level directive with a concrete message that provinces and sub-provincial level authorities needed to pay attention to HIV/AIDS.

The plan also illustrates a more dynamic image of HIV/AIDS in China, one that admits local diversity and uncertainty, and is based on model of human behavior that appears much less static than had been the case in the past. Thus, in reference to an evolving infection pattern, the plan said that 10,676 confirmed cases of HIV were reported in all provinces, but that the actual number could be over 300,000, and that by 2000, the number may be over 1.2 million (State Council of China 1998, 2). As transmission routes, it named drug use, sexual contact, and mother-to-child transmission and states that these are "all found in China" (State Council of China 1998, 2). In a reference to heterosexual spread, the plan talks about increasing numbers of STD cases and says that "HIV infection is increasing rapidly among the group of people who have multiple sexual partners and are not faithful" (State Council of China 1998, 2).

There is also a more dynamic view of the context in which HIV/AIDS spreads in China, and an admission, on the part of the government, of a certain degree of uncertainty and lack of control. Thus, the plan states that "China still lacks the capacity of stopping the prevalence of HIV/AIDS currently: some leaders of the governments and the related departments are not fully aware of the possibility and harm of HIV/AIDS' pandemic in China; the environment of prevention and control with a muti-sectoral [sic] collaboration and social participation has not yet been created; there is a lack of public knowledge of prevention . . . there is a shortage of expertise and a lack of effective experiences in HIV/AIDS and STDs prevention and control; and most doctors and nurses in the medical units and health agencies can not provide standard service in diagnoses and treatment for people with HIV/AIDS and STDs" (State Council of China 1998, 3). Also, the plan names previously unmentioned threats like rising HIV/AIDS epidemics in neighboring countries, the presence of a growing mobile population, drug use, and prostitution (State Council of China 1998, 3).

The Mid- to Long-term Plan represented an admission that HIV/AIDS could affect anyone in China, and a directive from the central level to the periphery to integrate prevention work (mainly education messages) at all levels. However, it also created a whole new question: given that HIV/AIDS existed in China, and that the country should act to stop it, what would be the appropriate way to do so? The existence of central-level directives did not automatically do away with disagreements over policy contents.

These tensions and uncertainties are illustrated in a public controversy about condom promotion that unfolded between the Chinese Center for Family Planning Publicity and Education and the State Administration of Industry and Commerce in 1999. In December of that year, the Chinese Central Television (CCTV) debuted China's first condom promotion spot, a 42-second message that explained the use of condoms for STD protection as part of a series of new efforts by the Center for Family Planning Publicity and Education to promote public awareness about sexual health and HIV/AIDS ("In a dramatic about-face, Beijing bans condom ads on China TV" 1999). On World AIDS Day, December 1, 1999, the State Administration of Industry and Commerce banned the spot, claiming that it violated the State Advertisement Law forbidding the advertisement of sex products ("In a dramatic about-face, Beijing bans condom ads on China TV" 1999).

An interesting debate about the distinction between a health message and a "sex message" unfolded in *China Daily*. Zhang Jian, the deputy director of

the Center, said that the advertisement "is not a commercial but a component of our program on AIDS prevention. Indeed we never intended to make
a commercial" (Meng 1999). Sun Guohua, a professor of legal philosophy
at Renmin University, argued that the ban was void because State Advertisement Law did not apply to this case—in an interpretation of administrative
discretion that assigns agency to the periphery when central directives are
considered unclear, he said, "it is unreasonable to cite a law governing com-
mercials to ban the condom announcement that is apparently for the benefit
of the public . . . The administration should follow the country's policy when
there are grey areas in current legislation" (Meng 1999). The ban was later
lifted, but for the time being, a deadlock remained.[9]

If a disagreement existed at the central level over what constituted a successful HIV/AIDS prevention and control, this was all the more true at the
local level. The Mid- to Long-Term Plan did not offer any financial support
to provinces to implement its recommendations, and at the time, central-
level HIV/AIDS funding still amounted to only about 15 million CNY (Wu
et al. 2007). This may explain in part why approaches to HIV/AIDS at the
provincial and county levels initially varied widely. Some provinces started
by passing laws to curtail the rights of HIV-infected individuals; for example, Chengdu City introduced a law mandating any individual employed
in a hotel, in a restaurant, at a travel agent, or in a public bath to get
tested for HIV and to leave their job in case of a seropositive result (United
Nations Joint Programme on AIDS (UNAIDS) 2002, 30). Other localities
took much more open approaches to the problem, and contradicting policies
could coexist within the same province.

The second half of the 1990s also saw an intensification of international
cooperation on HIV/AIDS within China, with an increasing flow of resources
coming from Europe and the United States. According to the Ministry of
Health, the total amount of aid received in 1985–1996 was US$ 17.4 million
("China spends nearly 5.6 million US dollars on HIV/AIDS prevention"
1998). In 1994, the EU invested 2.4 million Euro for prevention and training ("China-EC AIDS, VD treatment training programme launched" 1994).
In 1996, the World Bank and the Chinese Ministry of Health co-initiated
an HIV/AIDS prevention program that targeted Yunnan, Beijing, Tianjin,
and Shanghai and was initially supported with US$ 10 million ("Project
launched to prevent HIV/AIDS among Chinese" 1996). In 1997, UNDP
gave US$ 1.9 million for four years for supporting China in preventing and
controlling HIV/AIDS ("UN to help China fight AIDS" 1997). Other agencies that had been conducting projects in China on HIV/AIDS since the early
1990s include the United Nations Children's Fund (UNICEF), the United
Nations Educational, Scientific and Cultural Organization (UNESCO), the

European Union, the Australia Government's aid programs (AusAID), and the Ford Foundation (see Settle 2003, 64). The WHO gave US$ 14 million in 1998–1999 ("WHO to increase technical assistance" 1998).

Substantial parts of this money went into provincial-level programs, especially in southern provinces. For example, by 1997, international organizations including the WHO, UNDP, and UNAIDS had spent US$ 1.6 million for supporting HIV/AIDS control in Yunnan (Zhu 1997). In 1998, the United Nations Population Fund (UNFPA) provided US$ 14 million to support reproductive health and family planning programs for rural Chinese women, which included a major HIV/AIDS prevention component (Settle 2003, 65).

Between vague directives from the central-level, local initiative and cooperation with foreign agencies, a matrix of experimentation came to exist in a small number of hard-stricken localities. In the following, I will report on research conducted in Pingxiang, a county in one of the cities in Guangxi province that faced HIV epidemics in their injection drug user populations (also see Szlezák and Howitt 2004, 2005a, 2005b). This city's response to HIV/AIDS illustrates the challenges that officials at the sub-provincial level faced in addressing HIV/AIDS before 2001. It also illustrates the resources, local and foreign, that they could potentially draw on. Most importantly, it makes visible some of the ways in which ideas about HIV/AIDS, its presence in China, the need to prevent it, and the question of what policies were adequate became transported and accepted in the local context in the late 1990s.

In Pingxiang, a town on the border between the province of Guangxi and Vietnam, public security officials were first alerted to HIV/AIDS in 1996, when officials from the neighboring Vietnamese province reported that they had been observing growing HIV rates in the local injection drug user population. On testing a sample of individuals in Pingxiang injection drug users, public security officials had found an infection rate of more than 15 percent. To Pingxiang's newly instituted director of public health, this was enough to convince him that HIV/AIDS should be addressed in that population. However, the idea that Pingxiang's general population may be in danger of contracting HIV/AIDS did not immediately follow from this information.

At the prompting of a high-ranking official at the provincial-level CDC in Nanning, who had been monitoring the spread of HIV/AIDS in the province, the health director attended a UN meeting on HIV/AIDS in Bangkok in neighboring Thailand in 1997. He recalled visiting a famous temple that had been turned into a shelter for AIDS patients: "I thought, 'I have to prevent this from happening in Pingxiang.'" Thus, seeing HIV/AIDS affect elements of the general population in a neighboring Asian country convinced the county-level official that HIV/AIDS could threaten Pingxiang's general population in the same way. Similarly, officials related to me that seeing prevention programs carried out in Thailand or Vietnam did at least as much or more to persuade public health and police officials that certain interventions may be a good idea than warnings from the World Health Organization that compared China to Africa or Europe.

With continued support from the provincial level, Pingxiang's health and CDC officials embarked on a journey to educate first themselves about HIV/AIDS and later to get the county to address HIV/AIDS. This required delicate political work. Pingxiang's mayor and party secretary, who had the convening power necessary to set county policy and who could induce other departments to cooperate, resisted the idea. The health director said:

> We were absorbing as much information from outside as possible. At the same time, we were trying to get the other government officials to absorb it as well. We kept repeating the issue, over and over and over again . . . There was a great reluctance to accept reality, a reluctance to learn.
>
> (Szlezák and Howitt 2005a)

The high infection rates in injection drug users served as the basis for a series of initially covert interventions in that population. Health officials showed great imagination, initiative, and creativity in targeting injection drug users and prostitutes. An unofficial cooperation arrangement was made with the police to enable health personnel to target these groups. This involved the (unofficial) institution of days on which drug users and prostitutes could move in the town without fear of being arrested. The head of the health department initiated his own prevention policy by personally teaching injection drug users how to sterilize injection equipment:

> I told them [the injection drug users], if you have to use drugs, don't do it intravenously. If you have to do it intravenously, don't share needles. If you have to share needles, clean them overnight. To the police, this looked like we were teaching them how to use drugs.
>
> (Szlezák and Howitt 2005b, 7)

This quote illustrates the basic tension between the public health and law enforcement tenets that was present in China at the time. Chinese authorities maintained relatively severe policies against injection drug use. At the same time, they first unofficially and later (after 2002) officially endorsed public health policies that aim to decrease HIV infection during drug use (harm reduction interventions). Thus, the provision of sterile injection equipment was piloted in a project in Southern China starting in 1999 (Hammett et al.

2003; Hammett, Norton, et al. 2005). The local authorities tolerated these and other approaches as pilot programs that could be blamed on "the foreigners" in the case that they were regarded as having failed.[10] Hammett et al. have proposed a number of reasons for the fact that the Chinese authorities maintained severe policies against injection drug users while at the same time first unofficially and later officially endorsing harm reduction: the appearance, within the Chinese administration, of "champions" for such policies; a generally pragmatic attitude and willingness to consider public health evidence; an increasing degree of cooperation across sectors (including public health, police); the influence of the SARS epidemic; and increasing pressure from international partners to conform with the international HIV/AIDS paradigm (Hammett et al. 2008).

Introducing prevention efforts targeting Pingxiang's general population was even more delicate work. Local officials feared that admitting the presence of HIV/AIDS in the county would harm trade and economic development. After a year of persistent lobbying, the health officials received the go-ahead from the county's top officials, but were essentially told "whatever you do, don't mention Pingxiang." In the period between 1998 and 2000, the officials managed to engage all local departments, from the TV station to the Youth League and Women's Federation in general education efforts, as previewed in the 1998 Mid- to Long-Term Plan, but without ever making public any information about the presence and extent of HIV/AIDS in the county.

Even with the support from the city's mayor and party secretary, engaging other city departments was difficult. Again, the example of neighboring countries worked as a method of demonstration. The following account of the local representative of the All China Women's Federation (ACWF) after a visit to Thailand illustrates this:

> The department of health told us that AIDS prevention should be a main part of our work. At the beginning, we did not really understand this. I took this to be . . . a favor to the department of health, but not a part of the ACWF's regular work. The turning point was a study tour to Thailand. On that visit, I understood that women's involvement in preventing HIV/AIDS is very important. Women's rights include health. Women in China are generally quite conservative, and the risk of infection is low; but there is still a risk to a woman's health [from the possibility that her husband is unfaithful], and this affects the whole family, so prevention is very important . . . Before I visited Thailand, I psychologically rejected the idea that we needed to think about HIV/AIDS. After the trip, I knew that our China, under its Communist leadership, should do things even better than Thailand . . . I was willing to join efforts in HIV/AIDS prevention as part of our own agenda.
>
> (Szlezák and Howitt 2005b, 4)

By the end of the 1990s, Pingxiang had a number of broad-based measures including sign posts on the border warning passing truck drivers of HIV/AIDS, peer education and health programs for local prostitutes, condom distribution in local hotels, and TV spots in the rural areas around Pingxiang (Szlezák and Howitt 2005a).

China's First Five-Year Plan for HIV/STD Control (2001–2005)

By 1999, leading Chinese scientists and health officials had become overtly critical of what they perceived as an insufficient drive and coordination on the part of the central government. *The New York Times* quoted a report underwritten by a group of leading Chinese health experts, stating, "owing to government indifference, AIDS prevention and control is gravely ineffective" (Rosenthal 2000c). The report also said that there may be a large epidemic among blood sellers. According to the article, experts pointed out the lack of agreement between health and nonhealth authorities over what measures should be taken, and Qiu Renzong, an eminent bioethicist at the Chinese Academy of Social Sciences, criticized the government for being stuck in patterns that belonged in the past:

> The central government does not seem to realize how serious this is. We have not yet had an effective risk reduction strategy, because some departments are very conservative. They think chastity is more important than condom use. They say that the only way to prevent HIV transmission is to rely on China's traditional values.
>
> (Rosenthal 2000c)

On World AIDS day 1999, Vice Health Minister Yin Daikui reported to the international community 15,088 official cases of HIV/AIDS and pointed to sexual intercourse and blood selling as major routes of transmission:

> China is in a grave situation and the tasks ahead are very hard and complicated, due to an enormous number of drug users and people with multiple sex partners, plus over 100 million transient people each year, and commercial blood-sellers, who are all vulnerable to HIV/AIDS.
>
> ("China has more than 400,000 HIV carriers: Health Ministry" 1999)

In 2000, the news of plasma donation-related epidemic in Central China broke. On October 28, *The New York Times,* citing a Beijing magazine called *China News Weekly,* reported that more than a dozen families were infected with HIV in a single village in Henan province's Shangcai county (Rosenthal 2000b). The article spoke of an "unreported, unrecognized AIDS epidemic" and explained that attempts to investigate the infections were being met with resistance from local authorities. Shangcai county, and especially the village of Wenlou, came to exemplify the plight of the former plasma donors in the press (see, for example, Sui 2001).

Chinese newspapers also started reporting on the Henan epidemic (see, for example, Rosenthal 2000a). In November, *Southern Weekend* in the Guangdong province wrote about AIDS in rural counties in Henan, estimating that more than 10,000 individuals were infected; *Huadong News*, a supplement to *China Daily*, for the first time mentioned the existence of "AIDS villages" in Henan, stating that important events had been "hidden," and condemned local authorities for suppressing information (Rosenthal 2000a).

The news of an extensive HIV/AIDS epidemic inside China, which could not be linked to a foreign source or to an obvious violation of socialist norms, was an important factor in changing the public image of HIV/AIDS. The Henan farmers were neither "foreigners" nor "perpetrators." They were unequivocally victims (in fact, they were considered "innocent" or "blameless" in China (Cao et al. 2006)). By the time World Aids Day 2000 arrived, the official tone started to shift. In a reference to the Central Chinese epidemic, *Renmin Ribao* reported that "what we understand about HIV is just the tip of an iceberg" and that World AIDS Day was "a chance to understand some things that have been hidden" ("China's once-hidden HIV fears now out in the open" 2000). The *China Daily* printed an article that read almost like a statement from the World Health Organization:

[HIV/AIDS] has become a public health hazard and a social problem... To prevent and control its spread is a matter that concerns the future of the nation. As the world's most populous country, China fully understands its arduous task and responsibility in controlling the AIDS epidemic.

("A total war against AIDS" 2000)

The *Southern Weekend* directly criticized the government for being slow in their response, arguing that it had taken China more than 10 years to come forth with a national-level strategy, while many other nations had established their national AIDS prevention plans within a period of 18 months after detecting their first case of HIV infection ("China's once-hidden HIV fears now out in the open" 2000).

In June 2001, at the same time that the United Nations convened a General Assembly Special Session on HIV/AIDS in New York, China's Ministry of Health published the country's first Five-Year Plan on HIV/AIDS, entitled "China Plan of Action to Contain, Prevent and Control HIV/AIDS (2001–2005)" (United Nations Joint Programme on AIDS (UNAIDS) 2002, 33).

The document placed unsurprising emphasis on the need to ensure blood and blood products were safe and to raise HIV/AIDS awareness in the general population. It also stated the goal of reaching HIV/AIDS patients with diagnosis, treatment, and care services—by the end of 2002, the plan said, at least 50 percent of HIV/AIDS patients in China were to have access to "community and home care"; in addition, it specified targets for increasing the availability of standardized services including HIV/AIDS diagnosis, treatment, counseling, prevention, and care in county-, city-, and township-level hospitals. With the new plan came a marked, if still insufficient, increase in the central budget for AIDS prevention and care, from 15 to 100 million CNY (United Nations Joint Programme on AIDS (UNAIDS) 2002, 33).

Not surprisingly, UNAIDS criticized the plan on several levels (United Nations Joint Programme on AIDS (UNAIDS) 2002, 33–34). First, the agency pointed out that China's targets fell short in aspiration of the goals that UNGASS had endorsed—for example, the target that information and services necessary to prevent HIV/AIDS should be made available to 90 percent of young adults by 2005. Second, it stated that the plan failed to include a strategy to address the plight of vulnerable populations, "including issues such as gender, migration and poverty." Third, it pointed out that there was no concrete information on how China was going to attain the set goals. And finally, UNAIDS argued, the plan failed to mention the crucial role that high-level political leadership and efforts to reduce discrimination associated with HIV/AIDS played in addressing the disease—in particular, the fact that China's UNGASS delegation was headed by the country's minister of health rather than by a more influential representative was interpreted as sign that China still looked at the epidemic through a narrow, mainly biomedical, lens.

Conclusion

In this chapter, I have traced the emergence of HIV/AIDS as a policy issue in China between 1985 and 2001. I showed that over time, HIV/AIDS was reframed from a foreigner's disease to a problem that could affect the general population. However, this did not automatically lead to agreement about which policies to institute. At the time China started applying for money to the Global Fund, its plan was fundamentally different from the global HIV/AIDS policy paradigm on which the Fund is built. No testing or treatment was being offered. Strong disagreements persisted, especially between health and nonhealth officials, about whether or not condom promotion and harm reduction measures were appropriate.

In the next chapter, we turn to the interaction between the Fund and China. We can now see why this interaction is worth studying as an example of the dealings between two different forms of governance. The Fund is based on a particular policy paradigm that is different from China's. It requires local actors to defer to scientific review at the global level. However, as this chapter has shown, many policies that are regarded as scientifically valid by the supra-national authority were considered incompatible with Chinese values and culture. Finally, the Global Fund also imagines a world in which the state at least partly abandons its planning mode and engages the grassroots levels in the design and implementation of health policy. Its rules require govern-ments to engage nonstate actors, civil society, and patients in making decision about policies and programs. This raises the question of how these differences played out in the interaction between the two entities. And what role does the Fund's institutional design play in the interaction between the two entities? What is the role of the local CCM and the global TRP? These questions will be the topic of the next chapter.

CHAPTER 6

The Fund's Impact on China's HIV/AIDS Policy

This chapter is devoted to the interaction between the Global Fund and China from 2002 to 2006. During that period, China's national HIV/AIDS policy changed fundamentally to become almost congruent with the global HIV/AIDS policy paradigm that served as the basis for the creation of the Global Fund. First, the government took responsibility for providing prevention and care to its citizens. Second, the 2006 Five-Year Plan to control HIV/AIDS embraced most policies that had previously been regarded as irreconcilable with Chinese values, including the provision of free sterile injection equipment and methadone to injection drug users.

The adoption of these policies required a fundamental change in the way the citizen is imagined in relation to the state. In the global HIV/AIDS paradigm, the citizen who is at risk of or infected with HIV is a target of as well as an agent in government policy. Governments are required to provide services to individuals even when they engage in behaviors that are illegal or considered undesirable. They are also required to actively engage the patient/agent in their response to HIV/AIDS. This was a departure from previous approaches to HIV/AIDS in China.

China's CCM process played an important part in this reframing. The combination of a source of substantial funding with a stakeholder inclusion process had powerful effects on the exchange between Chinese officials and led to a gradual acceptance of new policies. However, local experimentation played an equally important role. This chapter discusses implications for the question of how the Global Fund's institutional design plays out in the interaction between the global and the local level.

HIV/AIDS, "Harm Reduction," and the Patient/Agent

Chapters 2 and 3 of this book have discussed in detail the co-production of HIV/AIDS as a global health, human rights, and human security issue and the Global Fund as an institution to address it. In an influential editorial in the June 2000 issue of *Science*, UNAIDS director Peter Piot summarized the newly defined twenty-first-century response to HIV/AIDS as follows:

> Successful national programs appear to be characterized by at least seven features: the impact of all actors coming together under one powerful strategic plan; visibility and openness about the epidemic, including involving people with AIDS, as a way of reducing stigma and shame; addressing core vulnerabilities through social policies; recognizing the synergy between prevention and care; targeting efforts to those who are most vulnerable to infection; focusing on young people; and, last but not least, encouraging and supporting strong community participation in the response.
>
> (Piot 2000)

If we take this representation and hold it next to the set of HIV/AIDS policies that China had in place in 2001, we see that the two differ substantially. There was no alliance of "all actors" under one powerful plan, there was no assumption that testing and treatment are indispensable parts of a successful response (in fact, neither were available), and there was certainly no official endorsement for community participation.

The discrepancy becomes even more evident when we take a closer look at some of the social policies that Piot refers to. HIV/AIDS education and condom promotion, voluntary counseling and testing, and harm reduction programs—not a single one of the interventions that are commonly presented as being part of the public health consensus on how to approach HIV/AIDS—were widely accepted in China. While proponents existed for many of these measures, especially in the public health community, their implementation was still very controversial at the time.

It is worth pointing out that China was by no means unique in this. As Piot's same editorial reveals only a few lines later, the global HIV/AIDS policy paradigm that the HIV/AIDS community imagined was not at all universally accepted at the time:

> It is an accepted wisdom that responses to the epidemic must be based on solid scientific evidence. Unfortunately, too often science is neutralized by ideology when it comes to issues that are difficult for some members of society to accept. For example, harm reduction among injecting drug users, including needle exchange programs, has been shown in numerous studies to reduce the risk of HIV infection, and yet in most countries of the world such programs are not

supported by the government or are even against the law. Another critical area is sex education for school-aged children. Again, there is sound evidence from numerous studies that sex and life-skills education not only results in safer sexual behavior but also does not lead to earlier onset of sexual intercourse nor to increased sexual activity. So why do many school authorities deny their children access to life-saving sex education?

(Piot 2000)

Piot presents the non-acceptance of these policies as a "neutralization" of science by "ideology." Harm reduction and sex education for children are imagined as matters of science, not of values, culture, or society. The geographic location of the "numerous studies" that prove the validity of these interventions is regarded as irrelevant with respect to the question of whether or not they constitute universal (or local) knowledge.

Both needle exchange programs and sex education among youth are controversial until today. Thus, U.S. Congress bans the use of federal funds to support the provision of sterile needles and syringes to injection drug users (see Hammett, Chen, et al. 2005, 216). In 2006, UN Special Envoy on HIV/AIDS Stephen Lewis accused the Bush administration of "incipient neocolonialism," arguing that the abstinence programs that the Bush administration stipulates developing countries implement if they want to receive money from the US$ 15 billion President's Emergency Fund for AIDS Relief (PEPFAR) "had been shown not to work" ("US criticised for HIV aid effort" 2006). And in the context of a recent study that found one in four U.S. teenage girls had venereal diseases, the president of the U.S. Planned Parenthood Federation of America Cecile Richards reportedly said, "the national policy of promoting abstinence-only programs is a US$ 1.5 billion failure, and teenage girls are paying the real price" (Altman 2008).

In order to understand the fundamental resistance against these approaches, it is useful to look at the basic concept of the individual and their relationship with the state that underlies them. *Harm reduction* is commonly defined in the context of illicit drug use. In contrast to "supply reduction" and "demand reduction," which aim to reduce the level of injection drug use activity, harm reduction focuses on the short-term aim of reducing harm commonly associated with it—including the spread of HIV/AIDS (Hammett, Chen, et al. 2005). Implicit in this approach is the idea that many drug users will not or cannot end their addiction. Harm reduction programs typically encompass a variety of different behavioral interventions, including the provision of sterile needles and syringes, the provision of methadone to substitute for heroin use, education, testing services for HIV and other diseases, and

122 の Making of Global Health Governance

condom promotion (Hammett, Chen, et al. 2005). They also centrally rely on "peer education," or the idea that individuals that formerly (or currently) were part of an injection drug use community know best how to reach members of that group, and on the idea that the support and acceptance of the broader communities in which they operate is crucial to their success (Hammett, Chen, et al. 2005).

The concept of harm reduction represents a departure from law enforcement approaches to injection drug use. Law enforcement, in any society, operates with the goal to eliminate or at least curb illegal behaviors by punishing offenders. In this paradigm, the distribution of methadone or clean needles to injection drug users (and of condoms to prostitutes) is often seen as encouraging illegal or unwanted behavior. Many believe that the state should not take on such a role. Against these arguments, public health pragmatism argues that intensifying law enforcement measures drives at-risk individuals underground, thereby making them invisible to the state, which can in turn contribute to the spread of HIV/AIDS and other problems. Both law enforcement and public health approaches feel the need to make underlying social behaviors visible, but the former addresses the risk takers as "them," people who stand outside the domain of what the legitimate parts of society do or should tolerate, whereas the latter includes even aberrant behaviors as part of the "us"—segments of society that are entitled to attention, treatment, and care, no matter how destructive or deviant.

Although the term "harm reduction" is commonly used to refer to injection drug use, it can be seen as a broader principle in the context of HIV/AIDS. Since a vaccine against HIV/AIDS currently does not exist, behavioral interventions are at the center of its prevention. And since HIV/AIDS is sexually transmitted, these behavioral interventions operate in a controversial and little understood space. Sex education for young people, condom distribution in brothels, and methadone substitution for injection drug users are instances of the same principle in the sense that they target behaviors that are not well understood or not wanted by all or by some. And the reactions to these interventions have in common that in each case there is the fear that interventions by the state will encourage that unwanted behavior. Thus, sex education in schools is feared by some to induce promiscuity in teenagers, condom distribution among sex workers is seen as sanctioning prostitution, the provision of sterile needles and syringes is seen as encouraging heroine use, and so forth.

Embracing the global HIV/AIDS paradigm thus means embracing the basic principle of harm reduction (reduction of HIV transmission in certain behaviors, regardless of whether they are desirable and legal or not).

To generate a climate in which that happens, the HIV/AIDS community emphasizes individual agency of all of its target groups, regardless of how they became affected, as evident in the "non-moralizing" language that the HIV/AIDS community has so carefully developed to counteract stigma. Thus, *drug addicts* become *injection drug users, prostitutes* become *commercial sex workers, homosexuals* become *men who have sex with men,* and *HIV/AIDS patients* become *people living with HIV/AIDS.* In this carefully sanitized view of the world, the state has an obligation to provide health-related services to affected people even though they may be engaging in behaviors that some regard as undesirable (like promiscuity) and even when they are engaging in behaviors that are illegal (like prostitution and injection drug use).

It becomes clear that for China to adopt an HIV/AIDS policy like the Global Fund envisions it, much more was required than the resolution of a few technical controversies. It entailed a redefinition of the relation between the individual and the state, at least for the purpose of implementing HIV/AIDS policies. As the example of the "pornography drive" showed in Chapter 5, policies directed toward affecting sexual behavior in the general population had been aimed at reducing the level of sexual activity, not at changing the way people thought about protecting themselves against sexually transmitted diseases. Similarly, government approaches to injection drug use had traditionally been based on curbing injection drug use through the apprehension, detention, and re-education of drug users in state-run "detoxification" institutions (Hammett et al. 2008), not at reducing the rates of HIV transmission that happen in the context of injection drug use. Finally, policies directed at prostitution had in the past aimed to apprehend and re-educate prostitutes as aberrant individuals in military-like operations (referred to as "whore wars") (see, for example, Gil et al. 1996), not to reduce the level of HIV transmission through prostitution.

As Chapter 5 has also shown, some Chinese officials had changed their views on these issues. By the year 2000, the representations of sexual behavior, injection drug use, and prostitution were no longer as stark as the preceding paragraph may suggest. However, there was no widespread agreement on these questions. Most officials unfamiliar with HIV/AIDS regarded the basic idea behind the concept of harm reduction as plain "incompatible with Chinese values," as one informant from the Chinese Ministry of Health put it to me in an interview. But even health officials who were ready to experiment with these approaches were skeptical. Some thought that China was "different" or "unique" (Hammett et al. 2008), so that Western harm reduction approaches would not automatically apply to the Chinese context.

HIV/AIDS and Participation

The image of the individual that forms part of the HIV/AIDS policy paradigm has a second fundamental aspect to it. Beyond the idea that the individual is a recipient of government services even in the context of unwanted or illegal behavior, there is also the idea that the individual is not just an object of the state's response to HIV/AIDS, but as an active and indispensable part of it. The de-stigmatization referred to earlier in this chapter serves the aim of enabling all at-risk and affected groups to come out in the open and cooperate with the state in various ways to improve their own health and that of others. The "strong community participation in the response" to HIV/AIDS that Piot alluded to is part of the Global Fund philosophy and institutional design, which presents the participation of civil society as indispensable to its work, as explained in Chapter 4.

Again, this represents a departure from the way the relation between the individual and the state had been conceptualized in Chinese public health. Mao Zedong's STD campaign drew on community participation in the sense that the detection and treatment of STDs were declared "patriotic actions" in China's liberation from Western imperialism (see Cohen et al. 2000). However, the element of patriotism hinges on a stark us/them boundary, which was no longer present with respect to HIV/AIDS. Similarly, the apprehension of prostitutes and injection drug users for the purpose of re-education certainly does not rest on a view of these individuals themselves, their peers, or the broader community in which they interact, as a central part of a government response. How was the idea that civil society and patients should participate in the national response to HIV/AIDS thus going to play out in China?

China has become more amenable to the idea of nongovernmental activity. To achieve the goal of "balanced" growth for a comfortable (*xiaokang*) society by 2020, China's new leaders have become increasingly willing to pay attention to those unable to profit from China's impressive economic development; concomitantly, they have also become more open to the idea of nongovernmental activity as a way of complementing government capacity. As an example, the Chinese Ten-Year Plan for poverty alleviation clearly states that NGO support is needed if the implementation of government projects in resource-poor settings is to be effective (Saich 2006, 37). At the same time, senior Communist party leaders, true to the party's Leninist foundation, remain ambivalent about the development of an NGO sector and suspicious of organizations outside state control (Saich 2006, 37). This creates a situation where nongovernmental organizations operate in an ill-defined gray zone.

Three types of nongovernmental activity can be said to exist in China's HIV/AIDS policy scene. The first, and most easily defined type, is international NGOs. China Development Brief, a Beijing-based nongovernmental organization observing the development of civil society in China, lists about 20 foreign organizations that have been actively working on HIV/AIDS in China since the late 1990s, which include Doctors Without Borders, the Ford Foundation, UK Save the Children, and Population Services International (China Development Brief 2008). As mentioned in Chapter 5, international NGOs have played an important role as initiators of HIV/AIDS programs at a time when the disease was still politically taboo and resources to address it were essentially nonexistent. Many representatives (foreign and local) of these organizations later became members of the CCM.

The second category of nonstate actors is that of Chinese government-affiliated organizations. These organizations, also referred to by the paradoxical name of "government-organized NGOs" ("GONGOs") (see, for example, China Development Brief 2007), are formally affiliated with a ministry or a government agency and work on a wide variety of social issues, ranging from education and environment to health. China Development Brief, an NGO that observes China's civil society development, referred to them as "half-way house" to true NGOs, explaining that they perform a variety of functions in the space between the government and the growing number of more "real," citizen-initiated grassroots organizations that range from mediation with government agencies to more explicit policy advocacy (China Development Brief 2007). At its outset, the category of GONGOs included traditional Leninist "mass organizations," like the All China Women's Federation and the Chinese Youth League, which increasingly opened their ways of working in the direction of an NGO concept, and many new GONGOs have appeared in the 1980s and 1990s that are getting closer to the internationally accepted definition of an NGO (China Development Brief 2007). In the HIV/AIDS sector, an important example is the China Association for Sexually Transmitted Diseases and HIV/AIDS (China Development Brief 2007).

The third type of nonstate actors active in the HIV/AIDS space are grassroots civil society organizations. These are small organizations that have been initiated by individuals but are not affiliated with a government agency. One of the most prominent examples was Wan Yanhai's AIDS Action Project, which started operating in Beijing in 1993. Similarly, Thomas Cai created an HIV/AIDS support network called AIDS Care China in Guangzhou in 2001, after himself being diagnosed with HIV (He 2011). Over time, his organization expanded from one hospital in Guangzhou across several provinces, Guangzhou, Yunnan, Guanxi, and Hubei, and expanded its services from support and counseling to support throughout the treatment process and, in 2006, was awarded the UNDP's Red Ribbon Award, and international award to recognize effective community-based approaches to fighting HIV/AIDS (United Nations Development Programme 2006). Though AIDS Care China was not a formally registered organization, the Guangzhou health authorities collaborated with Cai in various efforts to reach local HIV/AIDS patients.[1] But overall, these organizations had been unofficially active, in an instable political climate, and with little access to financial and other resources.

Many Chinese health officials had become amenable to the idea of cooperating with informal NGOs in their efforts to combat HIV/AIDS. For example, health authorities in Guangdong province cooperated with Thomas Cai although his organization has no legal status in China.[2] Some officials have started to speak of "pure" NGOs—a term that seems to distinguish the grassroots NGOs from the GONGOs without using the word "real" (which would imply that the GONGOs are "fake").[3]

However, in 2002, there was still considerable uncertainty as to the rules and conditions under which China's public space was going to be expanded to include these new voices and actors. The government's ambivalence with respect to civil society actors continues to be evidenced in instances of arrests and intimidation of Chinese HIV/AIDS activists (see, for example, Rosenthal 2002; Di 2006). These restrictions have been reported to have risen in intensity in the run-up to the Beijing Olympics, as the January 2008 arrest of HIV/AIDS activist Hu Jia shows (Bristow 2008).

Evolving AIDS Policy: China's Applications to the Global Fund 2002–2006

China quickly became one of the most important recipients of Global Fund money. Of the US$ 470 million requested by China in six rounds for all three diseases the Fund covers, over US$ 340 million had been approved by February 2008; US$ 180 million of that money was for HIV/AIDS (The Global Fund to Fight Aids, Tuberculosis and Malaria 2008c). This is a substantial portion of the central government's budget. At the launch of the Five-Year Plan in 2001, central-level spending for HIV/AIDS prevention and control had only recently been augmented from CNY 15 million to CNY 100 million (United Nations Joint Programme on AIDS (UNAIDS) 2002). Over time, that budget increased to CNY 400 million in 2003 and then to CNY 800 million in 2004 and 2005 (Wu et al. 2007). This means that between 2001 and 2005, approximately US$ 310 million (CNY 2.2 billion) was spent on HIV/AIDS by the central government (Wu et al. 2007).

China's applications to the Global Fund reflect the evolution of the country's HIV/AIDS policy in that period. China began applying to the Fund from round one in 2002, on initiation and under the leadership of departments responsible for HIV/AIDS at the CDC and Ministry of Health. The Chinese Centers for Disease Control (CDC) are the main recipients of Global Fund money in all rounds. The proposal-writing process was thus closely intertwined with the formulation and development of national policy. Two of the applications were rejected, which reveals disagreements between the global authority and the local actor.

Between 2002 and 2006, the proposals changed along three principal dimensions. First, the target groups changed, shifting at first between injection drug users and plasma donors before being extended to the general population including youth and migrant workers. Second, the proposed policies changed, starting out with education, then adding free treatment and harm reduction and finally the fostering of HIV/AIDS NGOs at the grassroots levels. Finally, the level of responsibility the Chinese government was proposing to take for funding and sustaining HIV/AIDS interventions increased substantially in the course of the proposals.

Over the period of only four years, the official HIV/AIDS policy thus changed fundamentally to look very similar to the policy paradigm illustrated by the Piot quote. In the following, I will explain this evolution by tracing policies and propositions in each of the six proposals and putting them in context with general developments during that period.

Round 1 (March 2002): Injection Drug Users

China's first Global Fund application proposed HIV/AIDS prevention in injection drug users in Southern China. The proposal included educational interventions but no harm reduction policies. Submitted in March 2002, the proposal was rejected by the Fund's technical review panel (TRP) on the grounds that it was of "poor technical quality." According to one of the officials who oversaw the proposal-writing process at the CDC in Beijing, the TRP held that offering educational measures alone without also including harm reduction interventions was not congruent with state-of-the-art HIV/AIDS policy and would therefore not yield the desired results.

In the Fund's vocabulary, this is a case of the *global* expert disagreeing with the *local* expert. Chinese health experts are expected to defer to an imagined global scientific consensus according to which harm reduction is the correct policy design. As Chapter 5 has shown, Chinese experts, while willing to experiment with harm reduction, as evidenced by the existence of a small number of pilot programs in several provinces, were not convinced that harm reduction was broadly applicable to the Chinese context.

Round 2 (September 2002): Treatment for Former Plasma Donors

After this non-acceptance of the first proposal, the second proposal shifted the focus entirely away from injection drug users and toward former plasma donors. The CDC had hired a Chinese-American individual living in Beijing to support the grant-writing process. It was felt that the grant writing skills of a native English speaker would be helpful in producing a result that would pass the technical criteria of the Fund's TRP.

The application proposed to make antiretroviral treatment available to former plasma donors in Central China. The provision of treatment to victims of the *plasma economy* promised to be less prone to disagreements over technical matters than the approach to injection drug use. The approach also provided at least a partial response to growing controversy arising from the Henan HIV/AIDS epidemic. In January 2002, a decade after the initial infection of blood donors, the *South China Morning Post* reported that as many as 370,000 villagers were infected in Henan province and hundreds had died or were now entering the stages of "full-blown AIDS" (Settle 2003, 101). With no treatment in sight, some patients started efforts to draw national and international attention to their fate and their urgent need for treatment. For example, in an attempt to communicate that their predicament was not just an unfortunate coincidence but the result of an economic policy fostered by local government, they sent a video to the United Nations, to Chinese media, and to the Ministry of Health, which showed the passes for blood donation that the local authorities had provided them with ("HIV-scandal villagers' video plea" 2002). The *South China Morning Post* printed a quote from the video, with a patient declaring: "the Health Department promised us selling our blood was safe and their stamp is in my donation booklet. How could I get sick?" ("HIV-scandal villagers' video plea" 2002).

The plasma donor epidemic raised the obvious but uncomfortable question of whether or not the government (and which level of government) had any responsibility for treating these "victims." In May 2002, the China CDC announced a "national comprehensive care strategy" to ameliorate the situation of HIV/AIDS patients, with special centers to be established in affected regions, like Yunnan, and a national network of centers envisioned for the future (Zhang 2002a). However, there was no promise to make antiretroviral therapy available to all who needed it. The resources for the provision of antiretroviral treatment to Henan's HIV/AIDS patients were to come from the Fund.

In June 2002, a UNAIDS report entitled "China's Titanic Peril" criticized China's leadership for "insufficient political commitment," a general "scarcity of effective policies," and the absence of an offer to make therapy accessible for infected individuals (United Nations Joint Programme on AIDS (UNAIDS) 2002). The report aroused great anger in Beijing. For many Chinese (and arguably also Westerners) who had seen the 1997 Hollywood movie "Titanic," the title evoked an image of China as a giant sinking ship.[4] Chinese health officials rejected the report, saying it misrepresented the Chinese situation and did nothing to help China with its AIDS epidemic (Ang 2002).[5] A few days after the report came out, Wan Yanhai's *Aizhi Xingdong* (AIDS Action Project) was ordered to shut down after nine years of operating in Beijing. According to Wan, this happened because of the government's discomfort with the UN report and because of *Aizhi Xingdong's* criticisms of the government's slow response (Sui 2002a).

Only a few weeks later, in August, Wan was detained; news reports at the time immediately speculated that his detention was connected to his publishing of documentation of the Henan epidemic on the Internet (Saiget 2002; "Press Rights Group says China AIDS activist Wan Yanhai in detention" 2002), which later turned out to be true. Shortly thereafter, *Xinhua News Agency* reported that Wan had posted "illegally-acquired interior classified documents to overseas individuals, media sources and websites" ("Wan Yanhai released after confessing to crimes in leaking state secrets" 2002). The documents, which originated from the Henan health department, revealed that Henan officials had known about but publicly denied the HIV/AIDS outbreak since the mid-1990s (Rosenthal 2002). Again, the Chinese authorities were determined to keep the Henan situation invisible to the outside. But Wan's detention received international attention. According to the *New York Times,* his release came quickly and was the result of strong support from a variety of powerful stakeholders—thus, U.S. State Department officials expressed concerns regarding Wan's whereabouts during Jiang Zemin's U.S. visit, thereby signaling that his fate was of broader interest and had not gone unnoticed; at the same time, human rights organizations, academics, and diplomats were demanding his release, and his supporters protested in front of China's embassies in Paris and New York (Rosenthal 2002). Interestingly, the pending Global Fund application apparently played a substantial role in Wan's release: Chinese health officials received an unofficial message saying that they could not expect their US$ 90 million application to the Global Fund to be successful as long as Wan was being imprisoned, and sent an important signal to the authorities regarding the cost, actual and figurative,

China was incurring by keeping Wan imprisoned (see Rosenthal 2002). He was finally freed ("Wan Yanhai released after confessing to crimes in leaking state secrets" 2002) and soon thereafter, re-opened his organization in Bejing's Dongcheng district (Sui 2002c).

The second Global Fund proposal was submitted in September 2002. Despite the release of Wan, and efforts to professionalize the application by including international public health consultants in the writing process, the Fund rejected it again, for reasons of "technical quality." According to a member of the writing team at China CDC, the TRP held (in line with the statements in "China's Titanic Peril") that the Chinese government was not showing enough "political commitment" to the issue of HIV/AIDS in China. In particular, the TRP noted that in asking for coverage of the entire cost of first and second line antiretroviral treatment with Global Fund resources, the government was not providing enough of its own financial resources to ensure the project's sustained success.

This assessment generated indignation among many officials who were involved in the proposal design and writing process. Many felt that the Fund was "in no position" to judge the Chinese government's level of political commitment to a matter internal to China. Officials held that the Chinese proposals were of no lower technical quality than any of the other proposals the Global Fund had received. Instead, they insinuated, both rejections had been politically motivated by U.S. antipathies vis-à-vis China. Again, the Fund's "TRP-expert" disagreed with the "local expert." This time, there was a clear feeling of violation with the principle of non-interference in the doings of the sovereign state of China. There was great reluctance within the government on whether or not China should reapply and thereby risk another rejection.

Round 3 (May 2003): "China CARES"

The third Global Fund proposal was overshadowed by the unfolding of the severe acute respiratory syndrome (SARS) epidemic during winter and spring of 2002/2003. By exposing not only the weakness of the Chinese rural health system, but also the potential dangers of a rapidly spreading infectious disease for economic development, SARS did a great deal to make Chinese authorities more responsive to the idea of openly addressing HIV/AIDS (see, for example, Kaufman, Kleinman, and Saich 2006, 5). Several officials explained to me a general feeling that among the Chinese authorities that unless they acted in time, HIV/AIDS would soon turn into a similar catastrophe. SARS arguably also helped convince non-health officials of the importance of infectious diseases as an agenda item on the Chinese national policy agenda.

The proposal was entitled "China CARES," an acronym for "China Comprehensive Aids RESponse" (Country Coordinating Mechanism in China 2003) and a direct response to previous allegations that the Chinese government was insufficiently committed to combating HIV/AIDS inside its borders. China CARES was presented as a scale-up of one of a pilot program the CDC had initiated in late 2002 in Shangcai county. This program, which was modeled on the Brazilian experience of care provision in resource poor settings, had showed increased survival rates and improved health in the initial study group, so that the authorities had decided to scale it up as part of China CARES (Wu et al. 2007). Consultants in the application process presented the pilot program as proof that China was planning to scale up a program that already reflected a government commitment to helping its citizens. It promised to "accelerate and strengthen" the program in 56 counties (Country Coordinating Mechanism in China 2003, 20), so that within five years, more than 90 percent of HIV carriers (40,000 individuals) would have access to antiretroviral therapy, and 300,000 people would request Voluntary Counseling and Testing (Country Coordinating Mechanism in China 2003, 2). China CARES was to serve as a model that could then be scaled up in other areas (Country Coordinating Mechanism in China 2004, 3).

The proposal offered plenty of proof that its title was not merely cosmetic. First, the government proposed to cover the entire cost of first-line antiretroviral therapy as well as treatment for opportunistic infections. Second, government contribution to the project was projected to increase from US$ 5.2 million to US$ 30.4 million over five years, and the Ministry of Health had requested an additional US$ 12.5 million per year for it from the Ministry of Finance (Country Coordinating Mechanism in China 2003, 23). Finally, the proposal explained that the government had passed a number of measures enabling Chinese pharmaceutical companies to produce antiretroviral medication for the domestic market, as well as waiving tariffs on imported ARVs (Country Coordinating Mechanism in China 2003, 2), signaling political will to drastically reduce the cost of HIV/AIDS therapy.

The proposal was also an early hint to the later policy of "Four Frees and One Care" (discussed in further detail below) which promised to extend treatment to all patients in need: although its principal focus was on former plasma donors, the proposal stated that the government was exploring the possibility of offering free treatment to all Chinese in need (Country Coordinating Mechanism in China 2003, 23), and explicitly stated that "within the targeted counties" of China CARES, HIV/AIDS treatment and care services would also be made available to patients other than former plasma donors, "including drug users, sex workers and others, without discrimination" (Country Coordinating Mechanism in China 2003, 3).

Round 4 (April 2004): Harm Reduction

After the success of the third round the focus shifted back to drug users and prostitutes. The proposal targeted seven provinces and included all of the previously controversial policies—methadone substitution, needle exchange, and grassroots civil society intervention (Country Coordinating Mechanism in China 2004, 4). This may look surprising. However, it makes sense in light of the fact that since the failure of round one, the central authorities had changed the official policy on needle exchange and methadone substitution.

National policy directives had changed to include needle and syringe exchange in 2002, after two trials in Guangxi and Guangdong provinces had shown lower hepatitis C and HIV rates in their intervention arms (Wu et al. 2007). Interestingly, this practice was not officially sanctioned by the public security authorities; it was introduced under the term "needle social marketing," a term coined to avoid the connotation that needles were being given out for free and to suggest instead that the availability of sterile needles and syringes was being increased in combination with health and safety information (see Wu et al. 2007; Hammett et al. 2008). This local understanding of "social marketing" is interesting, as it seems to put more responsibility on the individual than the classic harm reduction paradigm postulates (the drug user is presented as taking the responsibility for actively seeking clean equipment).

With respect to methadone, the Chinese government introduced this practice in 2004, based on the perception that international evidence pointed to its usefulness in HIV/AIDS prevention (Wu et al. 2007). Hammet et al. observe that methadone substitution was more easily accepted than needle exchange – this was because it was seen as having "social benefits", such as a decrease in the incidence of crime, and an improved ability on the part of injection drug users to take part in social life; also, it was not seen as a form of direct support to drug users in the same ways as needle exchange (Hammet et al. 2008). In contrast to methadone, needle exchange does not reduce the use of heroine or the actual practice of injecting it.

In the Fund's terms, the local expert had come to agree with the global expert. However, we see that this did not happen through an automatic agreement about practices that had been sanctioned by global science, but after a local investigation of whether or not certain practices were applicable and appropriate to the local context. This process involved modification and adaptation.

Round 5 (June 2005): Preventing a Heterosexual Epidemic in China

The fifth round was targeted to preventing a heterosexual HIV/AIDS epidemic. This reflected broader changes in the government policy that had taken place in 2003. On World AIDS Day in December 2003, Premier Wen Jiabao had been the first Chinese head of state to publicly shake the hand of an HIV/AIDS patient on TV at Beijing Ditan Hospital, thereby signaling to the Chinese public that touching an HIV infected individual was safe (Wu et al. 2007). In the same month, the Ministry of Health had conducted a study in cooperation with UNAIDS which showed that HIV/AIDS rates were on the rise in China, with HIV/AIDS spreading from "high-risk populations to the general population" (China Ministry of Health & UN Theme Group on HIV/AIDS in China 2003).

Shortly thereafter, the government announced free antiretroviral treatment for all under the very Chinese title of "Four Frees and One Care." "Four Frees and One Care" was built on the programmatic foundation of China CARES and promised free antiretroviral drugs to infected individuals in the rural population and to poor urban patients, free counseling and testing services, free treatment for pregnant women and babies, and financial support for HIV/AIDS affected families (see, for example, Zhang et al. 2005). A State Council Working Group on AIDS (SCWGA) was created in early 2004, giving HIV/AIDS greater importance at the national level, and government spending increased from CNY 390 million Yuan in 2003 to CNY 810 million in 2004 (Kaufman, Kleinman, and Saich 2006, 31).

In line with this shift toward a greater emphasis on the general population, the fifth Global Fund proposal targeted groups that had heretofore received less attention: homosexuals, migrant workers, and people living with HIV/AIDS. The focus on these groups was justified by the argument that they were "likely 'bridge populations' that could contribute to a rapid growth and expansion of the epidemic in China" (Country Coordinating Mechanism in China 2005, 45). Like some of the preceding ones, this proposal also hinted at future policy changes. Specifically, it pointed out that the lack of a nongovernmental sector in China had "severely limited community involvement in HIV/AIDS despite clear recognition from central government leadership that such involvement is essential" (Country Coordinating Mechanism in China 2005, 44). In an attempt to solicit input from grassroots NGOs, a member of the proposal writing team placed a draft on the website of his NGO, China AIDS Info, where it was publicly accessible throughout the entire application process.

Round 6 (August 2006): Civil Society Action as Public Health Policy

The sixth Global Fund proposal introduced civil society engagement as an HIV/AIDS policy intervention in China. The proposal specifically proposed to target a range of societal groups that are considered hard to reach for authorities. These included prostitutes, homosexual individuals, injection drug users, out-of-school youth, and people living with HIV/AIDS. Three things make this proposal different from previous ones. First, it proposed the fostering of grassroots civil society organizations as the main way of reaching the target populations. Second, and for the first time in China's involvement with the Fund, the Principal Recipient of the grant was not going to be the China CDC, but the *China Association for STD and HIV/AIDS Control*, a government-affiliated organization registered at the Ministry of Civil Affairs (Country Coordinating Mechanism in China 2006), although this was later changed.[6] The Association was expected to distribute funding to other GONGOs, as well as to informal grassroots NGOs. Finally, the writing process was different. Round six was written in a "bottom up" process that solicited input from NGOs all over China. Again, registered as well as non registered NGOs were eligible to submit proposals.[7]

The Chinese Country Coordinating Mechanism

The previous section has discussed the evolution of China's HIV/AIDS policy in the context of the Global Fund application rounds. This section turns to the Country Coordinating Mechanism structure and role in that process.

Structure

China set up a country coordinating mechanism (CCM) at the time of the first Global Fund application round in 2002. Membership was given at the invitation of the Ministry of Health. Over time, more and more stakeholders began to understand the role of the new body and the substantial amounts of new resources for HIV/AIDS that were coming into China through it. Many different actors started applying to be members of the CCM, and were granted participation, until the CCM included 50 members.

At the time of its setup, the composition of the CCM differed substantially from the Global Fund's vision (Country Coordinating Mechanism in China 2004). In particular, the category "people's organizations" mainly includes the traditional Chinese mass organizations, which are organs of the Communist party. Similarly, the category "Chinese Non-governmental organizations" is also made up mainly of Chinese mass organizations as well as government-led organizations. Moreover, all categories, even the pharmaceutical companies, outnumber the two patient representatives from "Mangrove," a patient "self-help" group established in 2002, supported by the Ford Foundation (China Development Brief 2002a, 2002b). The composition of the CCM reflected the fact civil society in China's HIV/AIDS sector is relatively weak and inadequately represented (Table 6.1).

Table 6.1 The China CCM 2004 (Country Coordinating Mechanism in China 2004)

Category	Number	Examples
1. Government	13	Ministry of Health
		Ministry of Finance
		Ministry of Education
		Ministry of Public Security
		Ministry of Justice
		Ministry of Commerce
		State Family Planning Commission
2. People's Organizations	4	Chinese Youth League,
		All China Women's' Federation
3. Chinese Nongovernmental Organizations	5	Chin. Association of STD & Aids Prevention and Control
4. Academic Institution	5	Peking University, Health Science Center
5. International Multilateral Organizations	11	UNDP, UNAIDS, WHO, ILO, UNESCO, World Bank
6. Bilateral Organizations	6	DFID (UK), European Union
7. International Nongovernmental Organizations	3	SavetheChildren (UK)
8. Pharmaceutical representatives	5	GlaxoSmithKline, Shanghai Desano Biopharmaceutical Co.
9. Individual representatives	2	Patient representatives
Total	**54**	

In 2006, the CCM commissioned an external review. This review coincided with a reform of the Global Fund's guidelines for building a CCM, which newly required proof of a transparent process for electing a representative for each sector (The Global Fund to Fight Aids Tuberculosis and Malaria 2005b).[8] It was conducted by Bernard Rivers, director of "Aidspan," a New York based NGO that represents itself as a "critical friend" and "independent watchdog" of the Global Fund. The report evaluated the China CCM against the specifications given in the Fund's directions for the structure and functioning of CCMs (Rivers 2005). It recommended to down size the CCM to 19 members; to introduce a voting system for each of the sectors represented on the CCM; and to increase the representation of grassroots NGOs, and at-risk communities, (defined as injection drug users, prostitutes, former plasma donors and gay individuals (Rivers 2005)).

After the reform, the Chinese CCM was reduced to 18 members. Every sector or type of organization now had one or two representatives (except for the government). People living with HIV/AIDS were represented by Thomas Cai, the head of AIDS Care China. Many considered his membership on the CCM an improvement over previous patient representatives who were regarded as government-picked. Jia Ping, a Beijing lawyer and civil rights advocate was now also a member. He later started and led the China Global Fund Watch Initiative, an organization with the mission to be "an independent watchdog over the activities of the Global Fund" as well as to "promote the development of civil society in China" (China Global Fund Watch Initiative 2012). Jia Ping was also in charge of the 2007 election process for a civil society representative (see China Global Fund Watch Initiative 2009), which was regarded as transparent and well documented (see, for example, Huang 2011).

Overall, the government still had substantial power in the new CCM, but the balance among the different sectors had been adjusted to a setup in which NGOs and patients had more voice than before. Table 6.2 presents the CCM composition in 2006 (Country Coordinating Mechanism in China 2006).

Table 6.2 The China CCM in 2006 (Country Coordinating Mechanism in China 2006)

Type	Number	Examples
Government sector	6	Ministry of Health
		Ministry of Education
		Ministry of Justice
		State Food and Drug Administration
		Ministry of Finance
Academic/Educational Institutions	2	China Centers for Disease Control
		Research Center for West-China Development at the Central University for Minorities
Mass Organizations	1	Red Cross Society of China
Chinese Associations or Societies	1	Chinese Association of STD&AIDS Prevention and Control
Community-Based Organizations or other NGOs	1	Jia Ping (Ai Zhi Yuan Zhu Center for Health and Education)
Private Sector/ State-Owned Enterprises	1	North East Pharmaceuticals Group
International Multilateral Organizations	2	World Health Organization Beijing
		UNAIDS Beijing
International Bilateral Organizations	2	UK Dpt. For International Development (DFID)
		Embassy of the United States
International NGOs	1	Patient representative
People living with HIV/AIDS	1	Thomas Cai (China AIDS Care)
Total	**18**	

Effects

The CCM-process played an important role in the evolution of Chinese HIV/AIDS policy. In the following, I will use excerpts from interviews I conducted with Chinese officials, members of the CCM and civil society organizations in Beijing to illustrate some of the effects of the CCM process. First, the CCM process contributed to an increase in profile of HIV/AIDS with the Chinese government. Not only did it place within reach an important external source of funding, but it also required attendance and involvement on the part of many ministries with important roles to play in HIV/AIDS policy making, including the ministries of health, public security and finance. One CDC official who was in charge of the writing process in the first two rounds explained:

> Now I feel it's good [referring to the CCM-mechanism]. Before, I was worried, because all the time so many meetings, but now I think it's good. You can say anything [in the CCM meeting]. Also my government pays much more attention to this project [HIV/AIDS control].

The need to produce proposals with the degree of detail and intricacy required by the Fund created pressure on the authorities to release data and information on HIV/AIDS in China. As an NGO-representative explained:

> Anyone who reads the reports on [HIV/AIDS in] China can see there's a real lack of—there's a lack of data. And there's a lack of epidemiological data, social data, behavioral data, everything is—and, and if you live in China long-term you know that information is usually to some degree faked by local officials who are just filling out forms. In the proposal writing, we were pushing for more detail and data.

A second important function of the CCM was to bring to the table national and international stakeholders who usually do not directly interact with each other on HIV/AIDS policy. These parties included government bodies like the Chinese ministries of health, education, and finance; the pharmaceuticals sector; multilateral organizations like the World Health Organization and UNAIDS; bilateral programs like UK's DFID; and international NGOs like Save the Children UK. This led to intense discussion, debate and exchange of ideas which in turn served to further the HIV/AIDS policy agenda. As one interviewee from an international NGO explained, the CCM process served as a discussion forum to make decisions on the provision of free treatment, needle exchange and harm reduction:

> Round three and to some extent round four is starting to look like it will spur on the government to do a lot more. I mean this whole commitment to provide

free treatment, free testing, that came in part because of what was written in round three. So that you—that the writing of the proposal itself pushed the policy. When we were writing round four and—there was a lot of—there was a lot of argument about, uh, methadone and needle exchange. [the CCM process] exposes a lot of decision makers to new ideas and to much more progressive ideas.

Chinese health officials agreed with this assessment of the CCM as a forum for exchange of ideas. One Ministry of Health official explained China's decision to continue to apply after the first two rejections with the Fund' role in giving officials access to information about HIV/AIDS policy in other countries:

> We look at the Global Fund not just as a source of financial resources. We look at Global Fund as a provider of good incentive to encourage the government to be more open, more cooperative, and to have more chance to—to have good experience and lessons from other countries, from international societies. So this way we look at the Global Fund . . . We look at it as a good instrument to set up communication and dialogue to learn good experience from other countries. So that's why we still have strong interest, and we still have some proposals will be submitted to Global Fund in this time.

Third, by requiring the signature of every member of the CCM, the Global Fund application process created strong incentives for consensus finding among the parties. A CCM member compared it with other donor funding, emphasizing the Fund's unique design in requiring this kind of consensus finding as a prerequisite for funding:

> A lot of other application processes until the Global Fund came along are not really (.) uh, for the most part, are not sort of collective processes where you're trying to get something through a CCM and forward. I like that about the Global Fund. I mean I was a huge, I was extremely skeptical to begin with . . . but basically as part of a process I like when you throw that [the policy proposal] on the table with the guys from the ministry of treasury . . . you know, to go back three and four times and get fifty people [the CCM] to stand up and make presentations with a room of fifty people saying "this is where we're going with this money, what do you think?"

Almost all of the individuals interviewed for this project observed that applications to the Global Fund involved intense exchange and discussion and were sometimes marked by outright conflict between the participating actors—much more so than other aid application processes they were familiar with from their previous experience. One Chinese health official called it "a nightmare." Nevertheless, the CCM-process was rated overall positive by every single one of the respondents. One member of an international organization describes how his initial skepticism dissipated when he saw how the process created broad support for interventions that had been regarded as controversial:

> First, I thought, who dreamed up this nonsense that these guys [referring to China CDC] are the best people out there to run massive eighty million dollar projects? I had no idea. It's a ludicrous idea . . . it looked to me like it was wired to fail from the very beginning . . . but round 4, when we got into the process, and I, I saw how many people were being consulted, uh, we worked overtime to make sure people understood the responsibilities that they were accepting. Uh, it's an incredibly difficult way to work, but I came out of it saying, you now, anybody who got anything to say about this whole thing has had a chance to do it. If you haven't—if you haven't seen this, put it out there, had something to say about this, then it's like, you've been asleep. You, you can't come in and tell us "oh, well, I got this problem, I got that problem, blah, blah, blah—you know, the representation was all right there. It may be unwieldy and people don't understand the, the power of having an opinion, I mean, or didn't exercise it because they didn't understand, but I, I came out of it saying, 'we've got broad political support for doing some very good harm reduction in China.'"

Naturally, the prospect of funding, together with a deliberative procedure, provided a powerful incentive for cooperation on a range of different policies. As one NGO-member described the discussions in the application process:

> People said: look, if we write this [referring to harm reduction policies], we will get 50 million dollars—and it works, because look in these other countries.

The process also had direct and indirect effects on the participation of grass-roots civil society actors. On one occasion, during the writing of the third proposal, the patient representative refused to sign until the funding earmarked for grassroots NGOs was increased from 15 to 20 percent.[9] This individual had been seen as a "token representative" by some of the civil society actors who were at that point still excluded from the CCM.

The CCM-process also enabled those in the Beijing public health community who wanted to see this sector strengthened to propose policies and to get funding for this purpose. Once the money from round six arrived in China, local NGOs were created in response, even though observers at the time, careful in their assessment, asked whether this was the sign of true civil society growth or an effect of the availability of foreign funding (see, for example, China Development Brief 2008).

Outlook: China's Second Five Year Plan for HIV/STD Control (2006–2011)

In March 2006, the State Council issued China's first legislation directly aimed to HIV/AIDS control, the AIDS Prevention and Control Regulations, and a new Five-Year Action Plan to Control HIV/AIDS (2006–2010) (State Council of China 2006). The changes since the first Five-Year plan were striking. First, with the involvement of the Fund, the Chinese government took responsibility for treating HIV/AIDS affected citizens. Before 2003, only about 250 HIV/AIDS patients had received antiretroviral therapy in China (Cao and Lu 2005). By the end of 2005, free antiretroviral treatment had been made available to 19,000 people (Cao and Lu 2005). In 2007 that number reached 30,000 individuals from 800 counties in all 31 provinces (Wu et al. 2007; Zhang et al. 2007).

Second, all of the previously controversial policies were now on the official agenda—education, condom promotion, Voluntary Counseling and Testing, and free treatment. In addition, the plans also sets concrete targets for the scale-up of the harm reduction policies that had previously been so strongly rejected. Thus, the plan specifies that at least 70 percent of injection drug users in cities with a population of 500 addicts or more are to receive methadone treatment in "drug-maintaining clinics"; similarly, at least 50 percent of injection drug users are to have received clean needles, with the needle/syringe sharing rate reduced below 20 percent; and the condom use rate in high risk populations is to reach at least 90 percent (State Council of China 2006).

In a 2007 article in *The Lancet*, a group of authors led by Wu Zunyou, head of the National Center for AIDS/STD Control and Prevention at China CDC, discussed the turn-around in thinking that had happened in China. Speaking of initial "mis-steps," the article notes that containment and isolation had proven "ineffective":

> The development of a coherent policy was the result of a long and unsystematic process that involved initial mis-steps, considerable domestic and international education, debate, iterative trial-and-error learning, and scientific studies . . . In much the same way as other countries, traditional public-health methods of containment and isolation of infectious disease cases proved ineffective.
>
> (Wu et al. 2007)

Wu et al. go so far as to concede that these policies were probably counter-productive in that they drove at-risk populations under ground:

> Containment policies occurred in the context of rapid social and economic change, in which there were increases in drug use and changing sexual mixing

patterns. These early policies did little to stop transmission of HIV/AIDS in fact, they probably promoted concealment of risk activities and made identification of HIV reservoirs more difficult.

(Wu et al. 2007)

The article also positions NGO participation as an integral part of China's success. Interestingly, when referring to NGOs, "which are a new concept in China," Wu cites two news articles in *Xinhua News* and *China Daily* covering increasing NGO activity in China, rather than a government source (Wu et al. 2007).

Global Knowledge, Local Knowledge

The analysis of China's interaction with the Global Fund yields important insights into the interaction between the Fund and a local actor. We see that global and local knowledge and expertise are not easy to separate. "Local experts" in Beijing included Chinese and foreign individuals with public health training, HIV/AIDS patients, and public security officials. In addition, we have seen that individuals from different parts of China were likely to think differently about HIV/AIDS. Lines of nationality, culture and profession cut right across the body of "local experts" the Global Fund imagines.

We have also seen that local and global actors don't automatically defer to global science. The first two rounds of the Global Fund proposals illustrate how what the Fund's TRP presented as a matter of clear evidence was deeply cultural and political to many inside China. In each case, local practices were adopted after they had been piloted and tried out in China, and after officials had decided that they were apt for the Chinese context. Local experimentation and local adaptation preceded acceptance, sometimes with modification to policy design. Thus, needle exchange was presented as "needle social marketing" to prevent the impression that a practice that is considered undesirable is encouraged for free by the state.

This experimentation is likely to continue and to be necessary with respect to many aspects of HIV/AIDS prevention and care. In China's most Western province of Xinjiang, where an increasing injection drug use problem has developed in province's Muslim population, the success of needle exchange programs has depended on the inclusion of local religious leaders so as to generate a sufficient level of local community support (French 2006). This is likely a difference to other regions in China. Similarly, stigma may look different in different regions and subpopulations. In the case of former plasma donors, stigma was reported to result from the presence of HIV itself, not from activities the individuals engage(d) in (Cao et al. 2006). In other groups the relations between stigma resulting from the possible presence of HIV and stigma resulting from the activity that the individuals engage in have been more complex to define (Chan et al. 2007; Lau et al. 2007).

A similar example is that of voluntary counseling and testing. Many have warned that the scale-up of "VCT" services in China risks violating the rights of HIV positive individuals because, as one interviewee put it "the 'V' and the 'C' are often missing in Chinese VCT." China's 2006 proposal states that "access to confidential VCT is still limited" (Country Coordinating Mechanism in China 2006, 42). Test results are often not kept confidential, which is a violation of the individual's rights according to Western notions of privacy and can engender stigmatization of the individual. A study undertaken in several locations in China shows that the disclosure of HIV status to an individual is regarded as a family matter (Li et al. 2007). Thus, a family member is often informed before the individual itself. This leads to conflict between Confucian ideals of family connectivity and authority versus Western notions of individual rights and privacy (see, for example, Chen et al. 2007). In this situation, locally specific framings may be necessary to find common ground between the two positions.

One type of local knowledge that is part of the Chinese response does not appear in any of the Global Fund applications. The Five-Year plan specifies that "not less than 50 percent of AIDS patients satisfying the treatment criteria should have received the treatment of Anti-Retrovirus Drug (ARD) or Traditional Chinese Medicine (TCM)" (State Council of China 2006). However, TCM does not appear in any of the Global Fund proposals. The Fund draws the boundaries between what counts as rational and what counts as irrational differently from the way this boundary is drawn in China, where traditional and Western approaches to health and disease exist alongside each other.[10]

Conclusion

China's HIV/AIDS policy altered rapidly during the interaction with the Global Fund between 2002 and 2006. The interactive CCM-process pushed the boundaries of policy within the Chinese political system. It raised the profile of HIV/AIDS with the Chinese government. It brought diverse voices to the table and created exchange and discussion, as well as intense struggle over priorities and policies. It exposed local policy makers to new ideas. And because it not only gave people incentives to meet, but also required the approval of every member, the CCM-process created strong incentives for consensus building. Overall, the process was able to generate broad support for once controversial policies.

In the process, the CCM itself changed in size, composition and rules of operation, and became more inclusive and democratic over time. While it continues to be dominated by the Chinese health authorities, the introduction of voting rules has given more weight to representatives of grassroots civil society and people affected with HIV/AIDS. It also had direct and indirect empowering effects for Chinese grassroots civil society. It created a "slot" for civil society participation in the CCM, enabling patient representatives and civil society to push for their interests. And it empowered local public health actors who wanted to strengthen civil society, so that measures to strengthen grassroots organizations became part of the applications to the Fund.

The case study points to the intricacies of the relationship between the global and local, showing that it is not always easy to distinguish between "local" and "global" views. In the case of HIV/AIDS policies in China, opinions were divided not by lines of culture and nationality, but along professional lines. Acknowledging this diversity of local actors enables one to see that the CCM process enabled those who had been experimenting at the local level to bring the results into a wider forum.

The study also points to some down sides of the Fund's design. Thus, the scientific institutions that the Fund relies on for validation of local policies only accept knowledge that is created according to their own rules. The example of traditional knowledge shows that the Fund has not democratized knowledge in the same way as it has broadened its definition of health and disease, and of public health policy. As a consequence, some local perspectives get included, but not others.

CHAPTER 7

Public Health Policy Making in the Global Domain

This study set out to display the coming into being of a new global sector, with its rules, representations, and responsibilities, which is a puzzle in itself; to investigate how this sector differs from the existing system of international health governance, which is based on the representation of nation-states; and to illustrate how the new level of policy making relates to preexisting levels of governance. Using the Global Fund's emergence in the health domain, the study has demonstrated the co-production of an issue to be governed at a new scale (global HIV/AIDS, tuberculosis, and malaria) and of new governance structures to address it (the Global Fund).

The study illustrates that, crucially, the question of who is responsible for a sick human body is changing as new institutional forms are being created. "World responsibility" is emerging for some things, like HIV/AIDS, with the locus of responsibility shifting away from national governments and the multilateral agencies alone toward a broad arrangement of state and nonstate actors. But at the same time as new forms of governance are emerging, politics at the national level is ongoing. This study has provided a China-specific reading of how responsibilities are distributed between the local and global levels. National processes remain important as China domesticates HIV/AIDS, a disease that was initially regarded as a foreign problem. As the understanding of HIV/AIDS as a Chinese problem emerges and changes over time, and as China starts interacting with the Global Fund, the question becomes who takes responsibility for what in the interaction between the global authority and the local (national) level.

In this situation, the Fund's implicit normative commitment is to help national governments tackle their HIV/AIDS, tuberculosis, and malaria epidemics under the condition that they can show that they will make their citizens better-off in ways that are credible to international science. In this model, international science becomes the needle's eye through which all national health policy planning has to pass to receive global money. The responsibility for the initiation, design, and implementation of health policies still lies with the nation-state. However, the accountability of the global authority rests on and is defined by global technological standards, which become a surrogate for responsibility in the global domain. The study provides an ethnographic account of the interplay between China and the Fund, showing how global norms emerged through iterative proposal writing shaped by the Fund's institutional design (specifically, the Country Coordinating Mechanism), a hybrid process in which local, national, and global actors all had substantial input.

The Global Fund is one kind of global responsibility regime emerging alongside existing institutions. Other examples of responsibility regimes include the new "Product Development Partnerships," such as the Medicines for Malaria Venture or the Global Alliance for TB Drug Development, global partnerships that aim to redistribute the responsibilities for the development of drugs and vaccines in such a way as to yield health care interventions that cater to the needs of poor patients in developing countries rather than to those of patients in industrialized countries, or Western travelers to tropical regions. In a similar fashion, corporate social responsibility can be seen as an attempt to redefine the responsibilities of corporations in a way that transcends the mere adherence to laws and formal rules so as to include the furthering of the well-being of corporate customers and their larger communities. All of these examples represent new sets of rules that are redefining the interaction between state and nonstate actors.

The example of the Fund shows that the emergence of such alternative responsibility regimes alongside existing governance structures does not occur without friction. The very emergence of the Fund was the result of intense political struggles among existing actors and required the mobilizing of entirely new categories and representations, such that HIV/AIDS was reframed as a global security emergency. Once in existence and fully functional, the Fund challenged and continues to challenge the authority of national governments and multilateral institutions by introducing new rules into the domain, such as the requirement to include civil society in national responses against HIV/AIDS, tuberculosis, and malaria. Under earlier nation-based regimes, the main actors in health policy were national governments and the WHO. Under the Fund's regime, there are multiple participants at various levels, including local civil society, local branches of the WHO and UNAIDS, companies, and even a "global consumer" that the Fund attempts to reach through its Product(RED) campaign.

Contradictions remain. The absence of Traditional Chinese Medicine (TCM) in Global Fund applications discussed in Chapter 5 is one illustration of a larger problem—that of democratization, or who gets to participate in decision making over resource allocation. The Global Fund draws a particular boundary between what counts as rational and what counts as irrational, leaving little or no room for negotiation. This boundary is drawn differently in China, where many actors envision the use of TCM alongside Western medicine, despite the fundamentally different worldviews that underlie these two concepts of human health and disease.

More frictions are bound to arise along the lines of these changed patterns of participation, despite the Fund's attempts to cause as little disruption as possible. How these frictions are sorted out, and which of them will be constructive as opposed to destructive to the overall aim of providing health care to patients in developing countries, remains to be seen. However, the Fund's example holds important lessons for institution building in the global domain.

The study offers lessons with respect to three theoretical and practical domains. First, it yields insights into the dynamics of co-production as it investigates fundamental questions about the emergence of new knowledge along with new forms of governance. The study of tuberculosis, malaria, and HIV/AIDS shows that there are different ways in which an issue can come to be regarded as global. As we look at the co-production of health issues and health institutions over the course of the twentieth century, we witness the dynamic evolution of different forms of global governance. We see that the globalizing rationale has changed over time, first construed as "biomedicine," later as "human rights," and finally as "transnational-ness." With each change in the representation of health issues came a different institutional answer to the question of what needed to be done—first, vertical disease control programs, then the building of primary health care infrastructure in the context of the Alma-Ata movement, and finally, the idea that partnerships between multiple state and nonstate actors were the most effective way of tackling these issues. The debates over financing and funding described in chapters 2 and 3 represent transition points between these different institutional forms.

The Fund marked a departure from previous models of cross-sectoral health cooperation, which were based on national governments and the UN agencies as the main actors in health care provision. The establishment of the Fund illustrates how forming representations and identities is intimately intertwined with the creation of global institutions, with their shape, form, and convergence on certain ideas as constitutive of their mission and legitimacy. Thus, political struggles among multiple parties were necessary to make the international community abandon the view that the provision of antiretroviral therapy in developing countries to anyone who needed it was prohibitively expensive and technically infeasible. The issue of mother-to-child transmission and, more precisely, the fate of the child of the HIV-positive African mother served as a connecting thread between these multiple sites of contestation. A new identity had been created—that of a blameless victim of HIV/AIDS and at the same time a universal human patient.

The study also elucidates the relation between the global and the local, and the universal and the specific, particularly as regards the role of knowledge and expertise. The Fund and other players tend to conceptualize science as global and local knowledge as particular and place bound. This distinction serves to establish authority in the global domain, in which direct political legitimation (e.g., through representation by nation-states or elections) are frequently missing. Scientific knowledge is thus a crucial pillar on which global organizations build their authority to speak for issues of common concern. The example of South African president Thabo Mbeki's "flirtation" with alternative explanations of HIV/AIDS and the effectiveness with which organized science (as represented by the journal *Nature* and the group of scientists who authored the Durban Declaration) publicly challenged Mbeki illustrate the power of scientific institutions to confer authority in this new domain.

The study also yields insights into governance models for institutions and standard-setting in the global domain. The case of China suggests that solutions that come out of the context of "global science" do not automatically transfer across cultural and national boundaries. Rather, they have to make sense to local actors before they can be adopted, accepted, and implemented in national contexts. In these respects, the study suggests that a global authority should structure its governance and processes so as to leave room for the local experimentation and adaptation of policies. Put differently, global organizations should remember the adage "think globally, act locally" in designing their institutional practices.

The third set of insights this study provides relate to the work of the Global Fund itself. The study suggests that the Fund has accomplished important changes in global public health policy making. First, it has found a way to draw on existing players, to "reshuffle" them, and to make them work together under new rules. For example, developing country governments can now initiate programs with the help of local representatives of the technical agencies and of bilateral development agencies, thereby putting these representatives in the position of consultants to the government rather than as non-accountable actors who have donor money to give away. Similarly, representatives of government, civil society, and patients sit around one table in the CCM process, forced to discuss and resolve controversies about numbers, budgets, and national policies. Even though the Fund's model may not play out perfectly in reality and may be facing many challenges and problems (as difficulties in engaging civil society in China have shown), these are important changes in the dynamics between existing actors. The Fund has in this way created a new and potentially effective layer of policy making without causing major disruptions among existing actors.

The Fund has also managed to become an important force in setting international standards and norms. For example, it has induced the Chinese government to experiment with grassroots civil society as a central part of its HIV/AIDS interventions. China's HIV/AIDS policy is now congruent with prescriptions by UNAIDS and the WHO, a vision of global public health as relying on multiple actors, including patients, civil society, and the private sector. To the extent that the Fund was crucial in this process of harmonization, this can be regarded as a success in the Fund's terms—the dissemination of a particular view (defined by the WHO, UNAIDS, and other players involved in the creation of the Fund) of how HIV/AIDS policy should be made, globally.

Despite these harmonizing effects, the Fund has at the same time helped to preserve significant "local ownership" of programs and projects. Thus, while the outcome of the interaction between the Fund and China resulted in policies that were almost identical with UNAIDS's definition of best practice, these policies are implemented by the Chinese CDC, not by outside actors. They are regarded by Chinese officials as originating from China and owned by China. By letting local actors decide which policies to propose, and reacting to them in consecutive rounds, the Fund arguably adapted to the local pace of evolution in China's HIV/AIDS policy agenda. In this sense, the Fund is a relatively gentle means of harmonization across countries.

This brings us to the question of what kinds of powers the Fund has, and what its practices are for disseminating a global perspective. The Fund's powers are largely "reactive" in the sense that it does not actively seek out local actors nor implement projects on its own. Rather than working as a centripetal force effecting changes in a passive periphery of recipient countries, the Fund's evaluation and/or correction happens in response to the propositions of local actors, and these actors must actively initiate interactions with the Fund.

This also means that the Fund's effectiveness depends on specificities in the local situation. This study has shown that no matter how important the Fund may have been in accelerating and fostering changes in the Chinese HIV/AIDS policy agenda, these changes were not the consequence of the Fund's presence alone. Rather, they emerged from China's political and economic transformations at that period in history. A series of developments, including a change in China's political leadership, the spread of HIV/AIDS among former plasma donors, and the SARS epidemic, all played important roles in reshaping the Chinese leadership's image of HIV/AIDS and of health policy in general. With respect to China's HIV/AIDS policy, cooperation between local officials and international agencies and local experimentation was crucial to the adoption of the policies and interventions that are on the Chinese agenda today.

However, this does not mean that the Fund's reactive powers are not substantial. This study has shown that despite local stakeholder inclusion in the CCM, China's programs were not entirely and completely up to local experts. The Fund rejected China's proposals when its Technical Review Panel (TRP) regarded China's propositions as nonconforming with "global best practice" or as insufficiently backed by the national government. The Fund wields great influence by virtue of its financial might and institutional design. However, as far as this study is concerned, the Fund has neither imposed undesired policies on China nor erased valued local particularities in the Chinese context. Rather, it has facilitated and enabled the wider adoption of policies after they were tested out in local circumstances.

What features of institutional design particularly account for the Fund's successes? Reliance on science as the arbiter of local policy and the separation of technical review and resource allocation have worked to confer authority and have stabilizing effects—in much the same way that similar practices have historically worked in developed country contexts. These practices signal to applicant countries that their internal political situation need not influence the funding decision. And what counts as "best practice" in health policy is ultimately not decided by the Global Fund, but relies on a set of general standards that have been determined in the world's scientific and public health communities.

Especially important and encouraging is the Fund's apparent ability to learn and change its practices in the course of its own activities. Two years into its existence, the Fund changed the rules for the composition of CCMs to include voting, after concerns were raised that many CCMs had no true civil society representation. It is also illustrated in the Fund's swift reaction, in 2004, to the charge by health experts that funded projects for malaria did not comply with best practices.

The study also points to some potential weaknesses in the Global Fund's operational model. First and foremost, the study has shown that the Fund's success depends crucially on the participation of its partners. While the Fund has managed to create new rules for participation by existing actors, it is also creating new challenges for them. In the case of China, the work of local representatives of multilateral and bilateral organizations was crucial to the success of Chinese proposals. The local offices of the WHO, of bilateral development agencies, and of international NGOs contributed substantially to China's success, mainly in the form of human resources. Such active assistance could put considerable strain on these organizations, especially given that the advent of the Fund has created a whole wave of new national-level health projects that did not exist before.

Second, we have seen contradictions in the Fund's understandings of the relationship between science and politics. The "experts" that the Fund defines are not so easy to recognize in actual policy making. Lines of nationality, culture, and profession cut right across the body of "local experts" that the Fund envisions. Similarly, global "best practice" is not always as well defined or as universally accepted as the Fund's vision of global public health policy making at first suggests.

At the global level, the critique of the Fund by health experts in 2004 for not adjusting to changes in the standard for malaria therapy quickly enough is illustrative. While the Fund reacted rapidly to this claim and made changes in response, there is still a fundamental question of how the Fund and other global organizations will deal with this sort of challenge in the future. The question of who bears uncertainty and risk in the global domain remains unresolved, and is not likely to be settled soon.

Similarly, when the Fund's "global experts" (the technical agencies and the Fund's TRP) do agree on a best practice, local actors may not accept their conclusions as valid. This was evidenced in the fact that harm reduction policies were at first regarded as incompatible with Chinese values, although international health experts regarded them as scientifically proven interventions. Similarly, when the TRP makes decisions, they may not be accepted at the local level. We see that in China, the rejection of the first two proposals generated considerable indignation as well as the perception that the Fund's TRP was biased against China.

Finally, what can we learn from the Global Fund's example as other global issues emerge in varied policy domains? The Fund clearly offers an interesting and promising model for development aid. It takes no great stretch of the imagination to argue, for example, in analogy to HIV/AIDS, that children should be given access to primary and secondary school education through a "Global Fund for Education," so that every child can get access to schooling, regardless of nationality. Whether we will see this kind of development anytime in the near future remains unclear. As argued before, the Fund is one type of global responsibility regime alongside others, and whether its model will eventually be transferred to other domains is uncertain. But as the Fund responds to its own set of challenges, the biggest being sustained funding and demonstrated success in bringing treatments to patients, we must ensure that we learn as much as we can from the evolving experience of this innovative organization, which has emerged so rapidly but is already influencing health policy making in so many countries and regions.

Notes

Chapter 2

1. Initially, there was a dispute over whether or not public health officials had told the patient, Andrew Speaker, that he was contagious before he left United States or only after arrival at his destination in Italy: after he reentered the United States via Canada instead of coming back with an expensive professional evacuation flight, as the U.S. CDC had recommended, that dispute escalated into a debate over whether Speaker's behavior was punishable and whether or not public health officials should have forcibly restricted the patient's movements (Altman 2007; Grady 2007; Schwartz 2007).

2. The right balance between the horizontal and vertical approaches continues to be the focus of debate in public health, across communicable as well as noncommunicable diseases (Van Praag et al. 1991; Greenwood 1997; Bradley 1998; Atun et al. 2004; Victora et al. 2004; Anderson et al. 2006; Uplekar and Raviglione 2007). As an example, the Bill and Melinda Gates Foundation with its focus on generating new cost-effective health technologies can be regarded as a vertical organization. The Global Fund to Fight HIV/AIDS, Tuberculosis and Malaria was designed as a vertical program targeting humanity's biggest infectious killers, yet it is increasingly argued that these types of programs are less likely to succeed in the absence of functioning horizontal health infrastructure (Drager, Gedik, and Dal Poz 2006).

3. These are the eradication of hunger and poverty, the reduction of child mortality, the improvement of maternal health and the targeting of HIV/AIDS, malaria, and other diseases. See www.un.org/millenniumgoals (accessed May 24, 2008).

4. The fact that TB rates in industrialized countries started to decline in the mid- to late 1800s, and thus before the advent of antibiotics, has prompted a discussion about whether the worth of targeted (vertical) public health intervention is proven compared to much broader reforms changing behavioral norms in a given population (Fairchild and Oppenheimer 1998).

5. In response, WHO formulated a new plan, the "Strategic framework to decrease the burden of TB/HIV," that laid the basis for the joint intervention delivery in programs addressing HIV and TB together—the treatment of latent

TB infection was supposed to serve to reduce TB rates in HIV-positive individuals, while antiretroviral therapy was to strengthen immunocompetence in HIV/AIDS patients and thereby strengthen TB control efforts (Raviglione and Pio 2002).

6. Major outbreaks had happened among HIV-positive populations in New York, Florida (Miami), and Italy (Milan) (Iseman 1998).

7. Was it necessary to treat MDR-TB all over the world? Was it feasible? Paul Farmer and others made the argument that specialized treatment of MDR-TB needs to be made available to all affected patients, pointing to the "transnational nature of the modern TB pandemic" (Farmer et al. 1998). Critical voices held that global expansion of treatment for MDR-TB was too complicated and simply not cost-effective (Espinal et al. 1999; Smith 1999) and warned that focusing on MDR-TB would draw away resources from treating patients with nonresistant TB (Smith 1999).

8. According to Raviglione and Pio, DOTS received US$ 16 million in 1990, US$ 50 million in 1996, US$ 160 million in 1999, and US$ 190 million in 2000 (Raviglione and Pio 2002).

9. These were lack of political commitment, insufficient financing, human resources, management at the program level, quality and supply of TB drugs, and the general weakness of information systems (Raviglione 2003; World Health Organization 1998b, 2006). In addition to these general constraints, MDR-TB and the HIV/TB co-epidemics were considered special challenges.

10. This was to happen through the engagement of the 22 countries that bear 80 percent of the global TB burden (Lee, Loevinsohn, and Kumaresan 2002).

11. In 2000, the partnership convened the Stop TB Ministerial Conference in Amsterdam and issued the "Amsterdam Declaration to Stop TB"; in it, countries with high TB infection rates formally committed to reaching the global TB control targets the WHO had set (World Health Organization 2000a). Shortly thereafter, WHO re-centralized its TB sections into a new Stop TB department; according to Raviglione and Pio, this reflected the belief that success depended on a "clearly defined managerial approach" and a "more visible structure" (Raviglione and Pio 2002).

12. For a detailed description of the Global TB Partnership, see Lee et al. (Lee, Loevinsohn, and Kumaresan 2002).

13. For reasons yet to be fully understood, adult women in endemic areas lose their partial protection against the disease during pregnancy. For this reason, malaria is an important contributor to maternal mortality in endemic regions (World Health Organization 2007a).

14. For a detailed review of the history of malaria, see, for example, Carter and Mendis, "Evolutionary and historical aspects of the burden of malaria" (Carter and Mendis 2002).

15. An interesting account of the controversy between the League of Nation and the Rockefeller Foundation can be found in Stapleton's article "Lessons of History? Antimalarial Strategies of the International Health Board and the Rockefeller Foundation from the 1920s to the Era of DDT" (Stapleton 2004). For a detailed

history of malaria as a human disease, and of international approaches to its control, see Bruce-Chwatt and de Zulueta (1980).

16. By the 1940s, the foundation's antimalaria activities spanned locations in North America, South America, the Caribbean, Southern and Eastern Europe, and India (Stapleton 2004).

17. According to Stapleton, some studies conducted in the 1920s claimed that quinine could not permanently eliminate the parasite from the blood stream, prompting experts to reason that quinine was of limited use (Stapleton 2004).

18. For example, the eradication of malaria in Sardinia became the display case for the Rockefeller strategy, mainly by proving that eradication of malaria was feasible even if total elimination of the vector could not be achieved (Bruce-Chwatt and de Zulueta 1980, 172).

19. In 1948, Pampane had first suggested that malaria transmission could be interrupted (for the long term) through time-limited spraying of defined areas with DDT (Bruce-Chwatt and de Zulueta 1980).

20. With the exception of small programs in Ethiopia, South Africa, and Zimbabwe (Trigg and Kondrachine 1998).

21. For a detailed discussion of the campaign's results, see Bruce-Chwatt and de Zulueta (1980, 171–172).

22. For example, Gellman reports that for years, the Clinton administration, the U.S. CDC (Centers for Disease Control and Prevention), and USAID (United States Agency for International Development) resisted the idea that they should pay for large-scale testing in developing countries: the only exception to this was testing for the purpose of monitoring the spread of the epidemic; interestingly, and in violation to ethical norms for HIV/AIDS to be established later, the test results were not disclosed to those who had been diagnosed with HIV (Gellman 2000b).

Chapter 3

1. As this chapter will show, the Global Fund was created in response to the growing impact of the HIV/AIDS epidemic. Tuberculosis and malaria were added to the Global Fund's agenda only after its inception. In studying the Global Fund's emergence, this chapter therefore focuses on HIV/AIDS.

2. Activist pressure on pharmaceutical companies was at that time still focused on U.S. domestic needs (Gellman 2000d).

3. Gellman reports that Jonathan Mann, then director of the WHO's Global Aids Program, initiated thinking about the possibility of providing ARVs in developing countries on the basis of alternative pricing schemes as early as 1991 (Gellman 2000d), thus long before the founding of the WTO, or UNAIDS. According to his account, the WHO, under the lead of Director-General Hiroshi Nakajima, initiated negotiations with the top management of 18 pharmaceutical companies, which subsequently failed; among the main reasons was the concern about whether the large-scale provision of ART in infrastructure-poor settings was feasible or not.

4. For example, the AIDS Coalition to Unleash Power (ACT UP) was formed in direct response to Burrough Wellcome's launch of AZT, the first antiretroviral drug, in 1987 at a price of US$ 10,000 per patient per year (Gellman 2000d).

5. As the prices of pharmaceutical products are set separately in each country, the same drug can be sold at two different prices in two neighboring countries. In 2006, this issue has raised attention in the United States over the possibility that U.S. citizens buy drugs prescribed in the United States for a cheaper price in Canada (Jakes Jordan 2006; Lee 2006).

6. For example, according to Gellman, Glaxo proposed to introduce a regional pricing scheme in January 1997, which would have sold their Combivir at a minimum of US$ 2; but their local managers did not comply and could not be forced to reduce prices under the Glaxo management system (Gellman 2000d).

7. The subanalysis showed that if the HIV-positive individual had a high viral load, they were more likely to transmit the virus to their partner; circumcision of men had a protective effect on their partners (Quinn et al. 2000).

8. In 1999, South African Health Minister Tshabalala Msimang said that even if AZT was safe, distributing it to South Africa's 44 million HIV-infected individuals would require ten times what the government was currently spending on health care (Swarns 1999).

9. The *Nature* letter said: "No one . . . will reject the argument that there are times when the voice of those challenging the existing order must be heard. Your own colleagues have referred to the astronomer Galileo in this context. But this does not mean that all dissidents and 'heretics' can claim equal legitimacy merely on the basis of their persecution; democratically endorsed procedures exist through which their ideas can be put to the test, and viable heresies separated from those that, after close scrutiny, deserve to be placed aside . . . Politics has developed one set of such procedures: the ballot box, parliamentary debate and constitutional law. Science has developed its own, very different, set. Contrary to the impression given by your letter, science thrives on the ideas of heretics. But heretical hypotheses only become widely accepted in science if they prove useful and effective in understanding and interacting with the natural world. The peer-review system is little more than a way of speeding up the process of sorting out those ideas which have a greater chance than others of surviving intellectual scrutiny and testing through experiment . . . Those who have experienced rejection may choose to castigate this as 'censorship', but the vast majority of authors of the scientific papers that we reject on technical grounds accept the process as valid and necessary for the health of science." ("Dear Mr Mbeki . . . " 2000).

10. At the time, the South African government was contemplating the declaration of a national emergency to support the compulsory licensing for AIDS drugs (Swarns 2001b).

11. In April 2001, South African Health Minister Tshabalala Msimang said that the distribution of antiretroviral treatment was not a government priority ("South Africa's Failure on AIDS" 2001). It was not until March 2002 that the government started offering Nevirapine at pilot sites (Swarns 2001f); it took civil society action and a high court order for the program to be extended to the

whole country, and then later to victims of sexual assault (see Swarns 2001c; "World Briefing Africa: South Africa: AIDS Drug Sought" 2001; "World Briefing Africa: South Africa: Order to Distribute AIDS Drug" 2002; "World Briefing Africa: South Africa: AIDS Policy Change" 2002).

12. Communicated during a key note speech that Farmer held at a 2003 conference on HIV/AIDS in China at Harvard's John F. Kennedy School of Government.

Chapter 4

1. Some criticized this process as being in-transparent (Richards 2001; Poku 2002).

2. The Global Fund has since been experimenting with different ways to include funding for "health systems strengthening" (HSS) in its processes (see WHO Secretariat 2007): In Global Fund rounds 1–4, the applicants could apply for HSS expenditures in addition to the three stand-alone diseases, round 5 introduced a separate HSS component, and round 6 returned to a more strict framework, so that HSS funding could be obtained only in the context of activities necessary to support the specific disease components. However, the fundamental question continued to be a subject of debate (see, for example, Ooms, Van Damme, and Temmerman 2007).

3. This point of view was transmitted to me by many of the individuals I interviewed at the global as well as local (China) level.

4. A fifth important principle of the Global Fund's institutional design is that of *performance-based funding*. The principal recipient receives not the full grant but partial amounts in intervals, contingent on the fulfillment of certain performance indicators prespecified in the grant proposal. The monitoring and evaluation of the implementation are conducted by a local fund agent (LFA), an independent locally based auditor designated by the CCM (for detail on performance-based funding and the role of the LFA, see www.theglobalfund.org/en/about/structures/lfa/ accessed January 23, 2012).

5. The inception of the Fund prompted major discussions about the best way to engage the private sector. Reports that pharmaceutical companies were going to be represented on the Global Fund board (Poku 2002; Yamey and Rankin 2002) were quickly rejected by the Global Fund's Interim Executive Director Anders Nordstrom (Nordstrom 2002b). Instead, McKinsey & Company, a management consulting firm, was invited to fill this position (Nordstrom 2002b).

Chapter 5

1. In tracing the evolution of HIV/AIDS in China, Edmund Settle's *AIDS in China: An Annotated Chronology 1985–2003* proved to be a tremendously useful source of information. Settle documented epidemiological, political, legal, and public health developments related to HIV/AIDS in China as they appeared in major English-speaking national and international news sources between 1985 and 2003—for example, in *The New York Times, China Daily, Xinhua* news

agency, and the *South China Morning Post*. The *Chronology* was very useful to me in understanding the overall developments and in orienting myself on further sources of information.

2. In February 1987, Xinhua reported the death due to HIV/AIDS of a 13-year-old hemophilia patient who had received contaminated blood from a foreign source ("AIDS virus-infected patients taken good care of" 1987).

3. Of the 150,000 individuals who had been screened to that date, the majority were Chinese who had been abroad, STI patients, blood donors, foreigners, homosexuals, as well as prostitutes and their clients ("Risk groups to be eyed for AIDS" 1990).

4. The plasma economy entrepreneurs were referred to as "blood heads" (*xue tou*) (Zhang 2005).

5. Official numbers regarding the scale of the Henan HIV/AIDS epidemic continue to be hard to come by. Zhang reports that in 1997, a government investigation in one unnamed Henan village yielded infection rates of 18.2 percent among plasma donors and 11.1 percent among whole blood donors; in 1999, another investigation showed 25.0 percent and 9.1 percent, respectively; according to Zhang, these figures were officially part of the national ninth Five-Year Plan and were made public in the *Chinese Journal of Epidemiology* (Zhang 2005, 24).

6. Zhang recounts how he himself had learned about the epidemic in 1998, during his work in the infectious diseases ward at You'an hospital in Beijing. A group of farmers approached him unofficially, requesting to be tested for HIV/AIDS. After discovering, to his great surprise, that all of the individuals were HIV positive, Zhang frequently visited Henan province over a period of five years, visiting about one hundred villages, diagnosing and interviewing patients, and documenting the epidemic. He conducted his work with great personal courage and frequently ran into difficulties with his employer and with the central-level health authorities, after the Henan CDC complained that he was disrupting Henan province's HIV/AIDS prevention efforts. Zhang recounts connecting with Zeng Yi at the Academy of Sciences in Beijing, who was now working with Wang Shuping, shortly after his initial discovery, and both confirmed his findings (Zhang 2005).

7. In 1996, the Ministry of Finance initiated a special fund for HIV/AIDS. Starting at 5 million CNY, the contribution rose to 15 million between 1998 and 2000, and finally to 100 million CNY per year from 2001 onward (China Ministry of Health & UN Theme Group on HIV/AIDS in China 2003).

8. Also in 1998, the regulation on "Principles for HIV/AIDS Education and Communication," which was underwritten by nine different government departments, specified a basic approach to HIV/AIDS education, using the mass media, and condom promotion among risk groups (United Nations Joint Programme on AIDS (UNAIDS) 2002, 32). In what can be interpreted as the beginning of a move away from a pure law enforcement paradigm to one that acknowledges the importance of reducing stigma, the regulation specified that the mere possession of condoms should not be taken as proof that an individual was engaging in prostitution (United Nations Joint Programme on AIDS (UNAIDS) 2002, 32).

9. In June 2002, the National People's Congress called on the State Administration for Industry and Commerce to revoke the prohibition; the agency followed this call and subsequently announced the start of "public information advertisements" for preservatives in early 2003 (Zhang 2002b).

10. This was related to me by several health officials I interviewed in the province of Guangxi in 2003.

Chapter 6

1. Thomas Cai spoke about his work and the cooperation with local authorities at a workshop on HIV/AIDS and Social Policy in China held at the John F. Kennedy School of Government at Harvard in the summer of 2005.

2. See previous footnote.

3. This was related to me by an interviewee who had attended several Global Fund related meetings with high-ranking health officials, where the role of grassroots civil society in combating HIV/AIDS in China had frequently been discussed.

4. This was communicated to me by several interviewees in Beijing.

5. The Chairwoman for the UN Theme Group on HIV/AIDS in China, Siri Tellier, stressed that the report was intended to help raise awareness: "The Ministry of Health cannot bear the burden. Our main message is that others—including the UN, the public, the media—have to do more" (Ang 2002).

6. The Association later declared that it did not have the capacity to administer one Million USD, so the funds and process were subsequently handed over to the China CDC as Principal Recipient for distribution to grassroots NGO (China Development Brief 2007).

7. See www.china-aids.org/index.php?action=front&type=view_page&id=11 accessed 12 February 2008.

8. The Global Fund requires that "CCM members representing the non-government sectors must be selected/elected by their own sector(s) based on a documented, transparent process, developed within each sector" (The Global Fund to Fight Aids Tuberculosis and Malaria 2005b).

9. Personal communication by an NGO representative of the Global Fund application writing team.

10. Even if one stays within the paradigms of Western medicine, there are several ways in which TCM could play a role in the context of HIV/AIDS policy. First, one ore more TCM modalities (herbal medicine, for example) could have direct antiretroviral effects. The Artemisinin Combination Therapies (ACTs) which are currently recommended by the WHO as the standard in malaria therapy (World Health Organization 2006b), originally came out of TCM's vast repository of medicinal plants, and has been found to have anticancer effects in addition to its antimalarial activity (see Efferth 2007, for example). Zhang Ke argues that TCM should be systematically investigated for compounds with antiretroviral properties. He cites dramatically reduced death rates from one village in Henan where farmers have been taking an unspecified TCM regimen as an indication

that some TCM regimens may be effective against HIV (Zhang 2005, 32). Second, different TCM practices could amplify the effects of antiretroviral treatment, as some have claimed is the case for acupuncture (Zhou, Sun, and Wu 2000) or, as a matter of fact, interfere with them. In both cases, this would be valuable knowledge. Third, in the absence of any direct or indirect antiretroviral effects, TCM could matter in the management of antiretroviral therapy and its side effects by improving compliance and potentially softening side effects of ARVs. Patient compliance with drop-out rates of 8 percent are a serious problem in the implementation of China's antiretroviral programs (Wu et al. 2007), and it is not implausible that patients may be more inclined to continue their treatments if they are offered traditional medicine in addition to their antiretroviral therapy. On his trips to Henan, Zhang Ke observed that former plasma donors generally preferred TCM over Western drugs because they were perceived to have less side effects (Zhang 2005, 32). All of these approaches could make sense and, if combined with systematic study, would easily fit within generally accepted Western standards of evidence based public health and medicine.

Bibliography

"Action on AIDS in Africa." 2000. *The New York Times*, January 11, A24.

Aginam, Obijiofor. 2006. "Globalization of health insecurity: the World Health Organization and the new International Health Regulations." *Med Law* no. 25 (4):663–672.

"Aids can be Checked in China—Experts." 1987. *The Xinhua General Overseas News Service*, July 22.

"AIDS Drug Cost to Be Cut for Poor Women." 1998. *The New York Times*, March 6, 7.

"AIDS in South Africa." 2000. *The New York Times*, July 12, A20.

"AIDS Virus-Infected Patients Taken Good Care of." 1987. *Xinhua General Overseas News Service*, December 7.

Alnwick, D. 2000. "Roll Back Malaria—What Are the Prospects?" *Bulletin of the World Health Organization* no. 78 (12):1377.

Altman, Lawrence K. 1985. "The Doctor's World; AIDS Data Pour in, as Studies Proliferate." *The New York Times*, April 23, 3.

———. 1998. "AIDS Meeting Ends with Little Hope of Breakthrough." *The New York Times*, July 5, 1.

———. 1999. "The Doctor's World; In Africa, a Deadly Silence About AIDS is Lifting." *The New York Times*, July 13, F7.

———. 2000a. "U.N. Warning AIDS Imperils Africa's Youth." *The New York Times*, June 28, A1.

———. 2000b. "In Effort to Save Lives, South Africa Creates an Anti-AIDS Campaign that Minces No Words." *The New York Times*, July 9, 8.

———. 2007. "Experts Mostly Back Way U.S. Reacted in TB Case." *The New York Times*, July 5, 8.

———. 2008. "Sex Infections Found in Quarter of Teenage Girls." *The New York Times*, March 12.

Anderson, B. O., C. H. Yip, S. D. Ramsey, R. Bengoa, S. Braun, M. Fitch, M. Groot, H. Sancho-Garnier, V. D. Tsu, and Po Global Hlth Care Systems Public. 2006. "Breast Cancer in Limited-Resource Countries: Health Care Systems and Public Policy." *Breast Journal* no. 12 (1):S54–S69.

Anderson, Benedict. 1991. *Imagined Communities*. 2nd ed. London: Verso.

Anderson, Donna. 1987. "Peking Daily Cautions Against Western Threats of AIDS, Drugs." *The Associated Press*, February 4.

Ang, Audura. 2002. "China Officials Reject AIDS Report." *The Associated Press*, June 28.

Angell, Marcia. 1997. "The Ethics of Clinical Research in the Third World." *The New England Journal of Medicine* no. 337 (12):847–849.

———. 2000. "Investigators' Responsibilities for Human Subjects in Developing Countries." *The New England Journal of Medicine* no. 342:967–969.

Attaran, A., K. I. Barnes, C. Curtis, U. d'Alessandro, C. I. Fanello, M. R. Galinski, G. Kokwaro, S. Looareesuwan, M. Makanga, T. K. Mutabingwa, A. Talisuna, J. F. Trape, and W. M. Watkins 2004. "WHO, the Global Fund, and Medical Malpractice in Malaria Treatment." *Lancet* no. 363 (9404): 237–240.

Atun, R. A., N. Lennox-Chugani, F. Drobniewski, Y. A. Samyshkin, and R. J. Coker. 2004. "A Framework and Toolkit for Capturing the Communicable Disease Programmes within Health Systems – Tuberculosis Control as an Illustrative Example." *European Journal of Public Health* no. 14 (3):267–273.

Awuonda, M. 1995. "Swedes Support Unaids." *Lancet* no. 345 (8964):1563.

Balter, M. 2000. "Can WHO Roll Back Malaria?" *Science* no. 290 (5491):430.

Banerji, D. 1965. "Tuberculosis – A Problem of Social-Planning in Developing-Countries." *Medical Care* no. 3 (3):151–159.

Barboza, David. 2008. "China Orders New Oversight of Heparin, with Tainted Batches Tied to U.S. Deaths." *The New York Times*, March 22.

Bayer, T., and D. Wilkinson. 1995. "Directly Observed Therapy for Tuberculosis: History of an Idea." *Lancet* no. 345:1545–1548.

Behforouz, H. L., P. E. Farmer, and J. Mukherjee. 2004. "From Directly Observed Therapy to Accompagnateurs: Enhancing AIDS Treatment Outcomes in Haiti and in Boston." *Clinical Infectious Disease* no. 38 (Suppl 5):S429–S436.

Bill and Melinda Gates Foundation. 2008. *Bill and Melinda Gates Call for New Global Commitment to Chart a Course for Malaria Eradication* 2007 [cited February 27, 2008]. Available from http://www.gatesfoundation.org/GlobalHealth/Pri_Diseases/Malaria/Announcements/Announce-071007.htm?version=print.

Bloom, B. R., and C. J. L. Murray. 1992. "Tuberculosis: Commentary on a Reemergent Killer." *Science* no. 257 (5073):1055–1064.

PR Newswire 2006 "Bono and Bobby Shriver Launch (RED)TM in the U.S." October 13.

Bradley, D. J. 1998. "The Particular and the General. Issues of Specificity and Verticality in the History of Malaria Control." *Parassitologia (Rome)* no. 40 (1–2):5–10.

Breman, J. G. 2000. "Malaria Control Stymied in 2010, Mastered in 2025." *Bulletin of the World Health Organization* no. 78 (12):1450–1452.

Bristow, Michael. 2008. "Fears for Rights as Beijing 2008 Nears." *BBC News*, January 2.

Brooke, James. 1988. "Surge in AIDS Cases in Congo Could Be an Omen for Africa." *The New York Times*, January 22, A1.

Bruce-Chwatt, L. J., and J. de Zulueta. 1980. *The Rise and Fall of Malaria in Europe.* Oxford: Oxford University Press.

Brudney, K., and J. Dobkin. 1991. "Resurgent Tuberculosis in New-York-City – Human-Immunodeficiency-Virus, Homelessness, and the Decline of Tuberculosis-Control Programs." *American Review of Respiratory Disease* no. 144 (4): 745–749.

Brugha, R., and G. Walt. 2001. "A Global Health Fund: A Leap of Faith?" *British Medical Journal* no. 323:152–154.

Brundtland, G. H. 2002. "Address by Gro Harlem Brundtland," *Director-General, to the 55th World Health Assembly.* Geneva: World Health Organisation.

Bruno, J. M., R. Feachem, T. Godal, T. Nchinda, B. Ogilvie, B. Mons, R. Mshana, G. Radda, E. Samba, M. Schwartz, H. Varmus, S. Diallo, O. Doumbo, B. Greenwood, W. Kilama, L. H. Miller, and L. P. daSilva. 1997. "The Spirit of Dakar: A Call for Action on Malaria." *Nature* no. 386 (6625):541.

Buse, K., and G. Walt. 2000a. "Global Public-Private Partnerships: Part I—A New Development in Health?" *Bulletin of the World Health Organization* no. 78 (4):549–61.

———. 2000b. "Global Public-Private Partnerships: Part II—What Are the Health Issues for Global Governance?" *Bulletin of the World Health Organization* no. 78 (5):699–709.

Cao, X. B., S. G. Sullivan, J. Xu, Z. Y. Wu, and Cipra Project Team China. 2006. "Understanding HIV-Related Stigma and Discrimination in a 'Blameless' Population." *Aids Education and Prevention* no. 18 (6):518–528.

Cao, Y. Z., and H. Z. Lu. 2005. "Care of HIV-Infected Patients in China." *Cell Research* no. 15 (11–12):883–890.

Carter, R., and K. N. Mendis. 2002. "Evolutionary and Historical Aspects of the Burden of Malaria." *Clinical Microbiology Reviews* no. 15 (4):564–594.

Centers for Disease Control and Prevention. 1990a. "From the Centers for Disease Control. Outbreak of Multidrug-Resistant Tuberculosis—Texas, California, and Pennsylvania." *JAMA* no. 264 (2):173–174.

———. 1990b. "Outbreak of Multidrug-Resistant Tuberculosis—Texas, California, and Pennsylvania." *MMWR Morbidity and Mortality Weekly Report* no. 39 (22):369–372.

Chaisson, R. 2000. Report from Durban, South Africa. In *The Hopkins HIV Report.* Baltimore: Johns Hopkins AIDS Service.

Chan, K. Y., Y. Yang, K. L. Zhang, and D. D. Reidpath. 2007. "Disentangling the Stigma of HIV/AIDS from the Stigmas of Drugs Use, Commercial Sex and Commercial Blood Donation – A Factorial Survey of Medical Students in China." *BMC Public Health* no. 7:280.

Chandra, Rajiv. 1993. "China: No Sex Please, We're Chinese!" *Inter Press Service,* September 17.

Chang, H. E. 1995. "Antiretroviral Treatment Progress Reports from a European Conference." *BETA* no. 10 (2).

Chen, W. T., H. Starks, C. S. Shiu, K. Fredriksen-Goldsen, J. Simoni, F. J. Zhang, C. Pearson, and H. X. Zhao. 2007. "Chinese HIV-Positive Patients and Their

Healthcare Providers – Contrasting Confucian versus Western Notions of Secrecy and Support." *Advances in Nursing Science* no. 30:329–342.

Chen, X. S., X. D. Gong, G. J. Liang, and G. C. Zhang. 2000. "Epidemiologic Trends of Sexually Transmitted Diseases in China." *Sexually Transmitted Diseases* no. 27 (3):138–142.

"China's AIDS Experts Call for Education." 1994. *AIDS Weekly*, July 18.

"China's Homosexuals Urged to Come Out of Closet, Help with AIDS Education." 1993. *Agence France-Presse*, February 10.

"China's Once-Hidden HIV Fears Now Out in the Open." 2000. *ChinaOnline*, December 12.

"China-EC AIDS, VD Treatment Training Programme Launched." 1994. *BBC*, October 6.

"China Acts up to Crackdown on Sexually Transmitted Diseases." 1988. *The Xinhua General Overseas News Service*, May 31.

"China Aims to Keep HIV Infections Below 1.5 Million by 2010." 1998. *Xinhua*, June 30.

China Development Brief. 2002a. *Beginning to Get It*. [cited January 25, 2012]. Available from http://www.chinadevelopmentbrief.com/node/162.

———. 2002b. *HIV/AIDS Project Digest*. [cited January 25, 2012]. Available from http://www.chinadevelopmentbrief.com/node/162

———. 2007. *Editorial: "GONGOs" Are Here to Stay, But Need to Reform and Open up*. [cited February 2, 2008]. Available from http://www.chinadevelopmentbrief.com/node/1071/print.

———. 2008. *Directory of International NGOs (DINGO)* 2008 [cited March 27, 2008]. Available from http://www.chinadevelopmentbrief.com/dingo/Sector/HIV—AIDS/2-49-0.html.

"China Discovers First AIDS Virus Carrier." 1989. *The Associated Press*, November 1.

China Global Fund Watch Initiative. 2009. "Democracy in Bud." In *Report on the Election of Community-based Organizations and NGO Sector Representatives to the China CCM of the Global Fund 2006–2007*, ed China Global Fund Watch. Beijing. Available from http://www.cgfwatch.org/c9990/c10022.asp (accessed January 28, 2012).

———. 2012. *"About us"* 2012 [cited January 28, 2012]. Available from http://www.cgfwatch.org/c9990/default.asp.

"China has More than 400,000 HIV Carriers: Health Ministry." 1999. *Agence France Presse*, December 1.

"China Makes Efforts to Prevent Aids." 1987. *The Xinhua General Overseas News Service*, September 27.

China Ministry of Health & UN Theme Group on HIV/AIDS in China. 2007. *China Responds to AIDS: HIV/AIDS Situation & Needs Assessment Report* 1997 [cited October 27, 2007]. Available from www.unchina.org./unaids/ekey1.html.

———. 2003. *A Joint Assessment of HIV/AIDS Prevention, Treatment and Care in China*. Beijing.

"China Reports 194 Infected by AIDS Virus." 1990. *Xinhua News Agency*, February 8.

"China Says Argentine Died of AIDS." 1985. *The New York Times*, July 30.

"China Spends Nearly 5.6 Million U.S. Dollars on HIV/AIDS Prevention." 1998. *Xinhua News Agency.*

"China Steps up Anti-AIDS Measures." 1988. *The Xinhua General Overseas News Service*, January 29.

"Chinese Economists Join AIDS Research." 1992. *Xinhua General News Service*, December 28.

Chopra, M., and I. Darnton-Hill. 2004. "Tobacco and Obesity Epidemics: Not so Different After All?" *British Medical Journal* no. 328 (7455):1558–1560.

Chopra, M., S. Galbraith, and I. Darnton-Hill. 2002. "A Global Response to a Global Problem: The Epidemic of Overnutrition." *Bulletin of the World Health Organization* no. 80 (12):952–958.

Christakis, N. A., and J. H. Fowler. 2007. "The Spread of Obesity in a Large Social Network over 32 Years." *New England Journal of Medicine* no. 357 (4):370–379.

Cohen, J. 2006. "Global Health. Public-Private Partnerships Proliferate." *Science* no. 311 (5758):167.

Cohen, M. S., G. E. Henderson, P. Aiello, and H. Y. Zheng. 1996. "Successful Eradication of Sexually Transmitted Diseases in the People's Republic of China: Implications for the 21st Century." *Journal of Infectious Diseases* no. 174:S223–S229.

Cohen, M. S., G. Ping, K. Fox, and G. E. Henderson. 2000. "Sexually Transmitted Diseases in the People's Republic of China in Y2K." *Sexually Transmitted Diseases* no. 27 (3):143–145.

Cohn, D. L., F. Bustreo, and M. C. Raviglione. 1997. "Drug-Resistant Tuberculosis: Review of the Worldwide Situation and the WHO/IUATLD Global Surveillance Project. International Union Against Tuberculosis and Lung Disease." *Clinical Infectious Disease* no. 24 (Suppl 1):S121–S130.

Collins, H. 2000. "$100 Million AIDS Program for Botswana." *The Philadelphia Inquirer*, July 10.

Coluzzi, Mario. 1999. "The Clay Feet of the Malaria Giant and Its African Roots: Hypotheses and Inferences About Origin, Spread and Control of Plasmodium falciparum." *Parassitologia (Rome)* no. 41 (1–3):277–283.

Commission on Macroeconomics and Health. 2001. *Macroeconomics and Health: Investing in Health for Economic Development.* Geneva: The Commission on Macroeconomics and Health.

Connor, E. M., E. S. Sperling, and R. Gelber. 1994. "Reduction of Maternal-Infant Transmission of Human Immunodeficiency Type 1 with Zidovudine Treatment." *The New England Journal of Medicine* no. 331:1173–1180.

" 'Controversial' AIDS Film Fills Cinemas." 1989. *BBC Summary of World Broadcasts*, April 7.

Cooper, E. C. 1996. "Antiretroviral Combination Treatment Prolongs Life in People with HIV/AIDS." *AMFAR Report* (1996 January):1–5.

Copson, R. W., and T. Salaam. 2005. The Global Fund to Fight AIDS, Tuberculosis, and Malaria: Background and Current Issues. In *CRS Report for Congress (RL31712)*. Washington, D.C.

Country Coordinating Mechanism in China. 2008. *Global Fund Round 3 Proposal: "China CARES (China Comprehensive Aids RESponse) – A Community-Based HIV Treatment, Care and Prevention Program in Central China"* [The Global Fund to Fight Aids, Tuberculosis and Malaria – Round 5 AIDS Proposal] 2003 [cited March 27, 2008]. Available from http://www.theglobalfund.org/programs/countrysite.aspx?countryid=CHN&lang=en.

Country Coordinating Mechanism in China. 2004. *Global Fund Round 4 Proposal: "Reducing HIV Transmission among and from Vulnerable Groups and Alleviating Its Impact in Seven Provinces in China"* [The Global Fund to Fight Aids, Tuberculosis and Malaria – Round 5 AIDS Proposal] 2004 [cited March 28, 2008]. Available from http://www.theglobalfund.org/programs/countrysite.aspx?countryid=CHN&lang=en.

———. 2005. *Global Fund Round 5 Proposal: "Preventing a New Wave of HIV Infections in China"* [The Global Fund to Fight Aids, Tuberculosis and Malaria – Round 5 AIDS Proposal] 2005 [cited March 28, 2008]. Available from http://www.theglobalfund.org/programs/countrysite.aspx?countryid=CHN&lang=en.

———. 2006. *Global Fund Round 6 Proposal: Mobilizing Civil Society to Scale Up HIV/AIDS Control Efforts in China* [The Global Fund to Fight Aids, Tuberculosis and Malaria – Round 5 AIDS Proposal] 2006 [cited March 28, 2008]. Available from http://www.theglobalfund.org/programs/countrysite.aspx?countryid=CHN&lang=en.

Crossette, Barbara. 2001. "A Wider War on AIDS in Africa and Asia." *The New York Times*, April 30, A6.

Crothall, Jeffrey. 1993. "Health Official's Sacking Signals Beijing's Attitude to Homosexual Rights; AIDS: China Keeps the Gays in Line." *South China Morning Post*, August 15.

Daley, Suzanne. 1998. "AIDS Is Everywhere, but Africa Looks Away." *The New York Times*, December 4, A1.

———. 2000. "The World: AIDS in South Africa; A President Misapprehends a Killer." *The New York Times*, May 14, 4.

Davis, R. M., M. Wakefield, A. Amos, and P. C. Gupta. 2007. "The Hitchhiker's Guide to Tobacco Control: A Global Assessment of Harms, Remedies, and Controversies." *Annual Review of Public Health* no. 28:171–194.

"Dear Mr Mbeki. . . ." 2000. *Nature* no. 404 (6781):907.

Delta Coordinating Committee. 2001. "Evidence for Prolonged Clinical Benefit from Initial Combination Antiretroviral Therapy: Delta Extended Follow-up." *HIV Medicine* no. 2 (3):181–188.

Di, Lin. 2006. "Interview with AIDS Activist Hu Jia." *Radio Free Asia*, March 29.

Donnelly, John. 2001. "The World; Prevention Urged in AIDS Fight/Natsios Says Fund Should Spend Less on HIV Treatment." *The Boston Globe*, June 7, A8.

Drager, Sigrid, Gulin Gedik, and Mario R. Dal Poz. 2006. "Health Workforce Issues and the Global Fund to Fight AIDS, Tuberculosis and Malaria: An Analytical Review." *Human Resources for Health* no. 4:23.

"Drug Abuse, Prostitutes, Migration Cause AIDS Peril in China." 1993. *Agence France Presse*, September 9.

Druilhe, P. 2000. "Roll Back Malaria: Technically Feasible or Just Politically Correct?" *Bulletin of the World Health Organization* no. 78 (12):1453–1454.

Dunlap, D. W. 1996. "From AIDS Conference, Talk of Life, not Death." *The New York Times*, July 15, 7.

"The Durban Declaration." 2000. *Nature* no. 406 (July 6).

Dyer, O. 2006. "New Fund-Raising Scheme Fuses Profit with Philanthropy." *Bulletin of the World Health Organization* no. 84 (4):263–264.

Ebrahim, S., J. Garcia, A. Sujudi, and H. Atrash. 2007. "Globalization of Behavioral Risks Needs Faster Diffusion of Interventions." *Preventing Chronic Disease* no. 4 (2):article A32.

Eckholm, Erik. 1990. "Confronting the Cruel Reality of Africa's AIDS Epidemic." *The New York Times*, September 19, A1.

Eckholm, Erik, and John Tierney. 1990. "AIDS in Africa: A Killer Rages On." *The New York Times*, September 16.

Efferth, T. 2007. "Willmar Schwabe Award 2006: Antiplasmodial and Antitumor Activity of Arternisinin – From Bench to Bedside." *Planta Medica* no. 73 (4):299–309.

Elhaggar, S. 1993. "Treatment/Control of HIV Infection." *Arch AIDS Research* no. 7 (2):120–121.

Espinal, M. A., C. Dye, M. Raviglione, and A. Kochi. 1999. "Rational 'DOTS Plus' for the Control of MDR-TB." *International Journal of Tuberculosis and Lung Disease* no. 3 (7):561–563.

"Failure to Curb AIDS Can Sabotage Socialist Construction—Official." 1993. *Xinhua General News Service*, November 26.

Fairchild, A. L., and G. M. Oppenheimer. 1998. "Public Health Nihilism vs Pragmatism: History, Politics, and the Control of Tuberculosis." *American Journal of Public Health* no. 88 (7):1105–1117.

Farmer, P., F. Léandre, J. Mukherjee, R. Gupta, L. Tarter, and J. Y. Kim. 2001a. "Community-Based Treatment of Advanced HIV Disease: Introducing DOT-HAART (Directly Observed Therapy with Highly Active Antiretroviral Therapy)." *Bulletin of the World Health Organization* no. 79 (12): 1145–1151.

Farmer, P., F. Léandre, J. S. Mukherjee, M. Claude, P. Nevil, M. C. Smith-Fawzi, S. P. Koenig, A. Castro, M. C. Becerra, J. Sachs, A. Attaran, and J. Y. Kim. 2001b. "Community-Based Approaches to HIV Treatment in Resource-Poor Settings." *Lancet* no. 358 (9279):404–409.

Farmer, Paul J. Bayone M. Becerra, J. Furin, C. Henry, H. Hiatt, J. Y. Kim, C. Mitnick, E. Nardell, and S. Shin. 1998. "The Dilemma of MDR-TB in the Global Era." *International Journal of Tuberculosis and Lung Disease* no. 2 (11):869–876.

Fidler, D. P. 2003. "SARS: Political Pathology of the First Post-Westphalian Pathogen." *Journal of Law Medicine & Ethics* no. 31 (4):485–505.

"Fighting AIDS in Africa." 2001. *The New York Times*, February 25, A14.

Ford, N., and E. T'Hoen. 2001. "The Global Health Fund: Moral Imperative or Industry Subsidy?" *The Lancet* no. 358:578.

Forman, Lisa. 2008. " 'Rights' and Wrongs: What Utility for the Right to Health in Reforming Trade Rules on Medicines?" *Health and Human Rights: An International Journal* no. 10 (2):37–52.

"Former Ugandan dictator Idi Amin dies." 2003. *CNN.com*, 11/18 2007.

Forrester, John. 1996. "If p, Then What? Thinking in Cases." *History of the Human Sciences* no. 9 (3):1–25. doi: 10.1177/095269519600900301.

Foucault, Michel. 1979. *Discipline and Punish*. New York: Vintage Books.

Fox, W. 1958. "The Problem of Self-Administration of Drugs; with Particular Reference to Pulmonary Tuberculosis." *Tubercle* no. 39 (5):269–274.

———. 1962. "Self-Administration of Medicaments. A Review of Published Work and a Study of the Problems." *Bulletin of the International Union Tuberculosis* no. 32:307–331.

French, Howard W. 2006. "China's Muslims Awake to Nexus of Needles and AIDS." *New York Times*, November 12.

Frieden, T. R., P. I. Fujiwara, R. M. Washko, and M. A. Hamburg. 1995. "Tuberculosis in New-York-City – Turning the Tide." *New England Journal of Medicine* no. 333 (4):229–233.

Gellman, Barton. 2000a. "A Conflict of Health and Profit; Gore at Center of Trade Policy Reversal on AIDS Drugs to S. Africa." *The Washington Post*, May 21, A01.

———. 2000b. "Death Watch: The Global Response to AIDS in Africa; World Shunned Signs of the Coming Plague." *The Washington Post*, July 5, A01.

———. 2000c. "A Turning Point That Left Millions Behind; Drug Discounts Benefit Few While Protecting Pharmaceutical Companies' Profits." *The Washington Post*, December 28, A01.

———. 2000d. "An Unequal Calculus of Life and Death; As Millions Perished in Pandemic, Firms Debated Access to Drug; Players in the Debate Over Drug Availability and Pricing." *The Washington Post*, December 27, A01.

Gil, V. E. 1994. "Sinic Conundrum – A History of Hiv Aids in the Peoples-Republic-of-China." *Journal of Sex Research* no. 31 (3):211–217.

Gil, V. E., M. S. Wang, A. F. Anderson, G. M. Lin, and Z. J. O. Wu. 1996. "Prostitutes, Prostitution and STD/HIV Transmission in Mainland China." *Social Science & Medicine* no. 42 (1):141–152.

"Global Warming Disease Warning." 1999. *BBC News*, June 18.

Goldsmith, M. F. 1988. "Dec 1 Designated World AIDS Day: Message is 'Join the Worldwide Effort'." *JAMA* no. 260 (20):2969–2970.

Goldyn, Lawrence. 2000. "Africa Can't Just Take a Pill for AIDS." *The New York Times*, July 6, A25.

Grady, Denise. 2007. "TB Patient Says Officials Are Trying to Blame Him to Cover Mistakes." *The New York Times*, June 9, 11.

Gravelle, Hugh, Rowena Jacobs, Andrew M. Jones, and Andrew Street. 2003. "Comparing the Efficiency of National Health Systems: A Sensitivity Analysis of the WHO Approach." *Applied Health Economics and Health Policy* no. 2 (3):141–147.

Greenwood, B. 2000. "Malaria – First, Roll Back Expectations." *Bulletin of the World Health Organization* no. 78 (12):1453.

Greenwood, B. M. 1997. "What's New in Malaria Control?" *Annals of Tropical Medicine and Parasitology* no. 91 (5):523–531.

Hadlington, Simon. 1988. "Global Cooperation Pledged after First AIDS Summit." *Nature* no. 331:377.

Hale, P. 2001a. "Mission Now Possible for AIDS Fund – Adequate Support by the G8 Countries is Needed to Defeat this Global Killer." *Nature* no. 412 (6844):271–272.

———. 2001b. "Success Hinges on Support for Treatment." *Nature* no. 412:272.

Hale, V. G., K. Woo, and H. L. Lipton. 2005. "Oxymoron No More: The Potential of Nonprofit Drug Companies to Deliver on the Promise of Medicines for the Developing World." *Health Affairs (Millwood)* no. 24 (4):1057–1063.

Hammett, T. M., Yi Chen, Doan Ngu, Dan Dinh Cuong, Ly Kieu Van, Robert S. Broadhead, and Don C. Des Jarlais. 2005. "A Delicate Balance. Law Enforcement Agencies and Harm Reduction Interventions for Injection Drug Users in China and Vietnam." In *AIDS and Social Policy in China*, Joan Kaufman, Arthur Kleinman and Tony Saich. eds. Cambridge, MA: Harvard University/Asia Center.

Hammett, T. M., D. C. des Jarlais, Wei Liu, Ngu Doan, Tung Nguyen Duy, Hoang Tran Vu, Van Ly Kieu, and Meng Donghua. 2003. "Development and Implementation of a Cross-Border HIV Prevention Intervention for Injection Drug Users in Ning Ming County (Guangxi Province), China and Lang Son Province, Vietnam." *International Journal of Drug Policy* no. 14 (5/6):389–398.

Hammett, T. M., G. D. Norton, R. Kling, W. Liu, Y. Chen, D. Ngu, K. T. Binh, H. V. Dong, D. C. D. Jarlais, and D. C. Des Jarlais. 2005. "Community Attitudes Toward HIV Prevention for Injection Drug Users: Findings from a Cross-Border Project in Southern China and Northern Vietnam." *Journal of Urban Health-Bulletin of the New York Academy of Medicine* no. 82 (3):IV34–IV42.

Hammett, T. M., Z. Wu, T. T. Duc, D. Stephens, S. Sullivan, W. Liu, Y. Chen, D. Ngu, and D. C. D. Jarlais. 2008. " 'Social Evils' and Harm Reduction: The Evolving Policy Environment for Human Immunodeficiency Virus Prevention Among Injection Drug Users in China and Vietnam." *Addiction* no. 103: 137–145.

He, Na. 2011. "The NGO Leader: Support our Work." *China Daily*.

"Health Officials on Measures to Control Spread of AIDS." 1990. *BBC Summary of World Broadcasts*, December 5.

"Healthy Behavior Key to AIDS Eradication." 1990. *Xinhua General News Service*, November 9.

Hilts, Philipp J. 1990. "Leader in U.N.'s Battle on AIDS Resigns in Dispute over Strategy." *The New York Times*, March 17.

"HIV-Scandal Villagers' Video Plea." 2002. *South China Morning Post*, 09.

Holland, Lorien. 1994. "China Warns AIDS is Spreading." *United Press International*, November 29.

Hollingsworth, B., and J. Wildman. 2003. "The Efficiency of Health Production: Re-estimating the WHO Panel Data Using Parametric and Non-parametric Approaches to Provide Additional Information." *Health Economics* no. 12 (6):493–504.

Hopewell, P. C., B. Ganter, R. B. Baron, and M. Sanchez-Hernandez. 1985. "Operational Evaluation of Treatment for Tuberculosis. Results of 8–12-month Regimens in Peru." *American Review of Respiratory Disease* no. 132:737–741.

Hopewell, P. C., M. Sanchez-Hernandez, R. B. Baron, and B. Ganter. 1984. "Operational Evaluation of Treatment for Tuberculosis. Results of a 'Standard' 12-Month Regimen in Peru." *American Review of Respiratory Disease* no. 129:439–443.

Huang, Y. Y., G. E. Henderson, S. M. Pan, and M. S. Cohen. 2004. "HIV/AIDS Risk Among Brothel-Based Female Sex Workers in China: Assessing the Terms, Content, and Knowledge of Sex Work." *Sexually Transmitted Diseases* no. 31 (11): 695–700.

Huang, Yanzhong. 2011. The GlobalFund, China and Civil Society. In *Asia Unbound*: Council on Foreign Relations.

Ibrahim, Youssef M. 1998. "AIDS Is Slashing Population of Africa, U.N. Survey Finds." *The New York Times*, October 28, A3.

"In A Dramatic About Face, Beijing Bans Condom Ads on China TV." 1999. *ChinaOnline*, December 1.

"In Debate on AIDS, South Africa's Leaders Defend Mavericks." 2000. *The New York Times*, April 21, A7.

Individual Members of the Faculty of Harvard University. 2001. *Consensus Statement on Antiretroviral Treatment for AIDS in Poor Countries*. [cited February, 2012]. Available from http://www.cid.harvard.edu/cidinthenews/pr/PR_040401.html.

"iPod 'Slave' Claims Investigated." 2006. *BBC News*, June 14.

Iseman, M. D. 1985. "Tailoring a Time-Bomb. Inadvertent Genetic Engineering." *American Review of Respiratory Disease* no. 132 (4):735–736.

———. 1998. "MDR-TB and the Developing World – A Problem No Longer to be Ignored: The WHO Announces 'DOTS Plus' Strategy." *International Journal of Tuberculosis and Lung Disease* no. 2 (11):867–867.

Jakes Jordan, L. 2006. "Drug Imports from Canada Set to Be Eased." *The Associated Press*, September 22.

James, J. S. 2000. "South Africa HIV Dispute: Time to Stop and Think." *AIDS Treatment Newsletter*, April 7; (340):6–8.

Jamison, D. T., and S. Radelet. 2005. "Making Aid Smarter." *Finance and Development* no. 42 (2), http://www.imf.org/external/pubs/ft/fandd/2005/06/jamison.htm.

Jasanoff, Sheila. 2004. *States of Knowledge. The Co-production of Science and Social Order*. London: Routledge.

Kahn, Bill. 2000. "U.S. Offers Africa $1 Billion a Year for Fighting AIDS." *The New York Times*, July 19, A1.

Kamat, S. R., J. J. Y. Dawson, S. Devadatt, W. Fox, B. Janardha, S. Radhakri, C. V. Ramakris, P. R. Somasund, H. Stott, and S. Velu. 1966. "A Controlled Study of Influence of Segregation of Tuberculous Patients for 1 Year on Attack Rate of Tuberculosis in a 5-Year Period in Close Family Contacts in South India." *Bulletin of the World Health Organization* no. 34 (4):517–532.

Kanavos, P. 2006. "The Rising Burden of Cancer in the Developing World." *Annals of Oncology* no. 17:15–23.

Kapp, C. 2002. "Global Fund on AIDS, Tuberculosis, and Malaria Holds First Board Meeting." *Lancet* no. 359 (9304):414.

Kaufman, J., A. Kleinman, and T. Saich. 2006. "Social Policy and HIV/AIDS in China." In *AIDS and Social Policy in China*, Joan Kaufman, Arthur Kleinman and Tony Saich. eds. Cambridge, MA: Harvard University/Asia Center.

Kaufman, J., and J. Jing. 2002. "AIDS – China and AIDS – The Time to Act is Now." *Science* no. 296 (5577):2339–2340.

Kaul, I., and M. Faust. 2001. "Global Public Goods and Health: Taking the Agenda Forward." *Bulletin of the World Health Organization* no. 79 (9): 869–874.

Kenna, Kathleen. 2000. "AIDS Crisis Called Major World Threat." *The Toronto Star*, January 11.

Kerr, T., K. Kaplan, P. Suwannawong, R. Jurgens, and E. Wood. 2004. "The Global Fund to Fight AIDS, Tuberculosis and Malaria: Funding for Unpopular Public-Health Programmes." *Lancet* no. 364 (9428):11–12.

Kerr, Thomas, Karyn Kaplan, Paisan Suwannawong, and Evan Wood. 2005. "Getting Global Funds to Those Most in Need: The Thai Drug Users' Network." *Health Human Rights* no. 8 (2):170–186.

Kilama, W. L. 2000. "Roll Back Malaria in Sub-Saharan Africa?" *Bulletin of the World Health Organization* no. 78 (12):1452–1453.

Knox, Richard A. 1998. "AZT Price is Cut in Developing World." *The Boston Globe*, March 6, A4.

Kochi, Arata. 1991. "The Global Tuberculosis Situation and the New Control Strategy of the World Health Organization." *Tubercle* no. 72:1–6.

Koenig, S. P., F. Léandre, and P. E. Farmer. 2004. "Scaling-up HIV Treatment Programmes in Resource-Limited Settings: The Rural Haiti Experience." *AIDS* no.18 (Suppl 3):S21–S25.

Komatsu, R., D. Low-Beer, and B. Schwartlander. 2007. "Global Fund-Supported Programmes' Contribution to International Targets and the Millennium Development Goals: An Initial Analysis." *Bulletin of the World Health Organization* no. 85:805–811.

Krieger, L. 1998. "Past Optimism is Missing at Start of International AIDS Conference." *The Buffalo News*, June 28, 8A.

Kumaresan, J., P. Heitkamp, I. Smith, and N. Billo. 2004. "Global Partnership to Stop TB: A Model of an Effective Public Health Partnership." *International Journal of Tuberculosis and Lung Disease* no. 8 (1):120–129.

Lambert, M. L., and P. van der Stuyft. 2002. "Editorial: Global Health Fund or Global Fund to Fight AIDS, Tuberculosis, and Malaria?" *Tropical Medicine & International Health* no. 7 (7):557–558.

Latour, Bruno. 1987. *Science in Action: How to Follow Scientists and Engineers Through Society*. Cambridge, MA: Harvard University Press.

Latour, Bruno, and Steve Woolgar. 1979. *Laboratory Life: The Social Construction of Scientific Facts*. Beverly Hills: Sage.

Lau, J. T. F., K. C. Choi, H. Y. Tsui, and X. Su. 2007. "Associations Between Stigmatization Toward HIV-Related Vulnerable Groups and Similar Attitudes Toward

People Living with HIV/AIDS: Branches of the Same Tree?" *Aids Care-Psychological and Socio-Medical Aspects of AIDS/HIV* no. 19:1230–1240.

Lee, C. 2006. "U.S. to Stop Seizing Prescription Drugs Imported for Personal Use." *The Washington Post*, October 5.

Lee, J. W., E. Loevinsohn, and J. A. Kumaresan. 2002. "Response to a Major Disease of Poverty: The Global Partnership to Stop TB." *Bulletin of the World Health Organization* no. 80 (6):428.

Levy, N. C., R. A. Miksad, and O. T. Fein. 2005. "From Treatment to Prevention: The Interplay Between HIV/AIDS Treatment Availability and HIV/AIDS Prevention Programming in Khayelitsha, South Africa." *The Journal of Urban Health* 2005 Sep; no. 82(3):498–509. Epub 2005 Jul 27 no. 82 (3):498–509.

Lewis, Neil A. 2000. "Clinton Issues Order to Ease Availability of AIDS Drugs in Africa." *The New York Times*, May 11, 7.

Li, L., S. Sun, Z. Y. Wu, S. Wu, C. Q. Lin, and Z. H. Yan. 2007. "Disclosure of HIV Status is a Family Matter: Field Notes from China." *Journal of Family Psychology* no. 21 (2):307–314.

Long Martello, M., and S. Jasanoff. 2004. "Globalization and Environmental Governance." In *Earthly Politics. Local and Global in Environmental Governance*, S. Jasanoff and M. Long Martello. eds. Cambridge, MA: The MIT Press.

Lopez, Alan D., Colin D. Mathers, Majid Ezzati, Dean T. Jamison, and Christopher J. L. Murray. 2006. *Global Burden of Disease and Risk Factors.* New York, N.Y./Washington, D.C.: Oxford University Press and The World Bank (copublication).

Lu, C., C. M. Michaud, K. Khan, and C. J. L. Murray. 2006. "Absorptive Capacity and Disbursements by the Global Fund to Fight AIDS, Tuberculosis and Malaria: Analysis of Grant Implementation." *Lancet* no. 368 (9534):483–488.

Lurie, Peter, and Sidney M. Wolfe. 1997. "Unethical Trials of Interventions to Reduce Perinatal Transmission of the Human Immunodeficiency Virus in Developing Countries." *The New England Journal of Medicine* no. 337 (12):853–856.

Macartney, Jane. 1987. "Chinese Authorities Ban Sex with Foreigners to Stop AIDS." *United Press International*, September 29.

Maher, D., and P. Nunn. 1998. "Commentary: Making Tuberculosis Treatment Available for All." *Bulletin of the World Health Organization* no. 76 (2):125–126.

Mandelbrot, L., J. Le Chenadec, A. Berrebi, A. Bongain, J. L. Bénifla, J. F. Delfraissy, S. Blanche, and M. J. Mayaux. 1998. "Perinatal HIV-1 Transmission: Interaction Between Zidovudine Prophylaxis and Mode of Delivery in the French Perinatal Cohort." *JAMA-Journal of the American Medical Association* no. 280 (1):55–60.

Mann, Jonathan M. 1987a. "The World Health Organization's Global Strategy for the Prevention and Control of AIDS." *The Western Journal of Medicine* no. 147 (6):732–4.

———. 1987b. "AIDS – A Global Perspective." *Public Health Reports* no. 102 (5):693.

Markus, M. B., and J. E. Fincham. 2000. "Mbeki and AIDS in Africa." *Science* no. 288 (5474):2131.

Marseille, E., P. B. Hofmann, and J. G. Kahn. 2002. "HIV Prevention Before HAART in Sub-Saharan Africa." *Lancet* no. 359 (9320):1851–1856.

Martens, J. 2003. "The Future of Multilateralism after Monterrey and Johannesburg." In *Dialogue on Globalisation Occasional Paper No. 10*. Berlin: Friedrich Ebert Stiftung.

Mathers, C. D., and D. Loncar. 2006. "Projections of Global Mortality and Burden of Disease from 2002 to 2030." *Plos Medicine* no. 3 (11).

McCarthy, M. 2002. "A Brief History of the World Health Organization." *Lancet* no. 360 (9340):1111–1112.

McGregor, A. 1995. "Unaids Sets Preliminary Budget." *Lancet* no. 346 (8969):239.

McKenna, M. T., E. McCray, and I. Onorato. 1995. "The Epidemiology of Tuberculosis among Foreign-Born Persons in the United States, 1986 to 1993." *New England Journal of Medicine* no. 332 (16):1071–1076.

McNeil Jr., Donald G. 2001. "Indian Company Offers to Supply AIDS Drugs at Low Cost in Africa." *The New York Times*, February 7, A1.

————. 2008. "Gates Foundation's Influence Criticized." *The New York Times*, February 16.

Meng, Yan. 1999. "Condom Spot: Ad or Education?" *China Daily*, December 10.

Mons, B., E. Klasen, R. van Kessel, and T. Nchinda. 1998. "Policy: Biomedicine – Partnership Between South and North Crystallizes Around Malaria." *Science* no. 279 (5350):498–499.

"Mr. Gore and the AIDS Drugs." 1999. *The Washington Post*, June 24, A26.

Murray, Christopher J. L., and Alan D. Lopez. 1990. *The Global Burden of Disease: A Comprehensive Assessment of Mortality and Disability from Diseases, Injuries, and Risk Factors in 1990 and Projected to 2020*. Cambridge, MA: Harvard School of Public Health on behalf of the World Health Organization and the World Bank. Distributed by Harvard University Press.

Nabarro, D., and K. Mendis. 2000. "Roll Back Malaria is Unarguably both Necessary and Possible." *Bulletin of the World Health Organization* no. 78 (12): 1454–1455.

Nabarro, D. N., and E. M. Tayler. 1998. "The "Roll Back Malaria" Campaign." *Science* no. 280 (5372):2067–2068.

Nchinda, T. 1998. "Malaria: A Reemerging Disease in Africa." *Emerging Infectious Diseases* no. 4 (3):398.

Neville, Kathleen, Assia Bromberg, Ruven Bromberg, Stanley Bonk, Bruce A. Hanna, and William N. Rom. 1993. "The Third Epidemic – Multidrug-Resistant Tuberculosis." *Chest* no. 105 (1):45–48.

"Ninety-One More Drug Addicts Found Infected with AIDS." 1990. *The Associated Press*, July 17.

Nogueira, Susie. 2002. "Governments as Facilitators or Obstacles in the HIV Epidemic." *BMJ* no. 324 (January 26):184–185.

Nolte, E., and M. McKee. 2003. "Measuring the Health of Nations: Analysis of Mortality Amenable to Health Care." *British Medical Journal* no. 327 (7424):1129–1131.

Nordstrom, A. 2002a. "Global Fund for AIDS, Tuberculosis and Malaria." *Lancet* no. 359 (9317):1621–1622.

———. 2002b. "Global Voices on HIV/AIDS – Important Facts about Global Fund were Missed." *British Medical Journal* no. 324 (7344):1035–1035.

Nullis, Clare. 1995. "U.N. Tries to Overcome Infighting in Battle Against AIDS." *The Associated Press*, May 29.

Nye, Joseph S., and John D. Donahue. 2000. *Governance in a Globalizing World.* Washington, D.C.: Brookings Institution Press.

"Obesity 'Contagious', Experts Say." 2007. *BBC News*, July 26.

"Officials Say China Has No Time to Waste to Control AIDS." 1996. *Xinhua News Agency*, October 16.

Oliver, R. T. D. 2000. "Though HIV is the Main Cause of AIDS, Other Factors Play a Role." *Nature* no. 406 (August 17):673.

Omran, A. R. 2005. "The Epidemiologic Transition: A Theory of the Epidemiology of Population Change (Reprinted from The Milbank Memorial Fund Quarterly, vol 49, pg 509–38, 1971)." *Milbank Quarterly* no. 83 (4):731–757. doi: 10.1111/j.1468-0009.2005.00398.x.

Ooms, Gorik, Wim Van Damme, and Marleen Temmerman. 2007. "Medicines without Doctors: Why the Global Fund Must Fund Salaries of Health Workers to Expand AIDS Treatment." *PloS Medicine* no. 4 (4):605–608.

Pablos-Mendez, A., M. C. Raviglione, A. Laszlo, N. Binkin, H. L. Rieder, F. Bustreo, D. L. Cohn, C. S. B. Lambregts-van Weezenbeek, S. J. Kim, P. Chaulet, P. Nunn, and for WHO/IUATLD. 1998. "Global Surveillance for Antituberculosis-Drug Resistance, 1994–1997." *New England Journal of Medicine* no. 338 (23):1641–1650.

Pan, S. M. 1993. "China – Acceptability and Effect of 3 Kinds of Sexual Publication." *Archives of Sexual Behavior* no. 22 (1):59–71.

Parish, W. L., Y. Luo, R. Stolzenberg, E. O. Laumann, G. Farrer, and S. M. Pan. 2007. "Sexual Practices and Sexual Satisfaction: A Population Based Study of Chinese Urban Adults." *Archives of Sexual Behavior* no. 36 (1):5–20.

Parish, William L., and Sui Ming Pan. 2006. "Sexual Partners in China. Risk Patterns for Infections by HIV and Possible Interventions." In *AIDS and Social Policy in China*, Joan Kaufman, Arthur Kleinman andTony Saich. eds., 190–213. Cambridge, MA: Harvard University Asia Center.

PBS News. 2007. *Thabo Mbeki's Letter* 2000 [cited November 19, 2007]. Available from http://www.pbs.org/wgbh/pages/frontline/aids/docs/mbeki.html.

Perinatal HIV Intervention Research in Developing Countries Workshop Participants. "Science, Ethics and the Future of Research into Maternal Infant Transmission of HIV-1."*Lancet* no. 353:832–835.

Perlez, Jane. 1988. "Scientists from Western Countries Pressing for AIDS Studies in Africa." *The New York Times*, September 20, B5.

———. 1992. "Briton Sees AIDS Cutting Population in Parts of Africa." *The New York Times*, June 22, A8.

Petersen, Melody. 2001. "Abbott to Sell Low-Cost AIDS Drugs in Africa." *The New York Times*, March 28, C9.

Petersen, Melody, and Donald G. McNeil Jr. 2001. "Maker Yielding Patent in Africa For AIDS Drug." *The New York Times*, March 15, A1.

Pio, A. 1989. "Impact of Present Control Methods on the Problem of Tuberculosis." *Reviews of Infectious Disease* no. 11 (Suppl 2):S360–S365.

Piot, P. 2000. "Global AIDS Epidemic: Time to Turn the Tide." *Science* no. 288 (5474):2176–2178.

Poku, N. K. 2002. "The Global AIDS Fund: Context and Opportunity." *Third World Quarterly* no. 23 (2):283–298.

Poku, N. K., and A. Whiteside. 2002. "Global Health and the Politics of Governance: An Introduction." *Third World Quarterly* no. 23 (2):191–195.

Presidential AIDS Advisory Panel Report. 2007. Government of South Africa, 11/18 2007 2001 [cited November 18, 2007]. Available from http://www.info.gov.za/otherdocs/2001/aidspanelpdf.pdf.

"Press Rights Group Says China AIDS Activist Wan Yanhai in Detention." 2002. *Agence France Presse*, September 5.

"Project Launched to Prevent HIV/AIDS Among Chinese." 1996. *Xinhua News Agency*, May 17.

"Public Warned to be on Guard Against AIDS." 1989. *Xinhua General News Service*, December 1.

Quinn, Thomas C., Maria J. Wawer, Nelson Sewankambo, David Serwadda, Chuanjun Li, Fred Wabwire-Mangen, Mary O. Meehan, Thomas Lutalo, and Ronald Gray. 2000. "Viral Load and Heterosexual Transmission of Human Immunodeficiency Virus Type 1." *The New England Journal of Medicine* no. 342 (13):921–929.

Radelet, S., and B. Siddiqi. 2007. "Global Fund Grant Programmes: An Analysis of Evaluation Scores." *Lancet* no. 369 (9575):1807–1813.

Ramiah, I., and M. R. Reich. 2006. "Building Effective Public-Private Partnerships: Experiences and Lessons from the African Comprehensive HIV/AIDS Partnerships (ACHAP)." *Social Science & Medicine* no. 63 (2):397–408.

Ramsay, S. 2002. "Global Fund Makes Historic First Round of Payments." *Lancet* no. 359 (9317):1581–1582.

Raviglione, M. C. 2003. "The TB Epidemic from 1992 to 2002." *Tuberculosis* no. 83 (1–3):4–14.

Raviglione, M. C., P. Sudre, H. L. Rieder, S. Spinaci, and A. Kochi. 1993. "Secular Trends of Tuberculosis in Western-Europe." *Bulletin of the World Health Organization* no. 71 (3–4):297–306.

Raviglione, M. C., and A. Pio. 2002. "Evolution of WHO Policies for Tuberculosis Control, 1948–2001." *Lancet* no. 359 (9308):775–780.

Reichman, L. B. 1991. "The U-Shaped Curve of Concern." *American Review of Respiratory Disease* no. 144 (4):741–742.

Reinicke. 1997. "Global Public Policy." *Foreign Affairs* no. 76 (6):127–138.

Renaud, C., E. S. Byers, and S. M. Pan. 1997. "Sexual and Relationship Satisfaction in Mainland China." *Journal of Sex Research* no. 34 (4):399–410.

"Reversing the Failures of Roll Back Malaria." 2005. *Lancet* no. 365 (9469): 1439.

Richards, T. 2001. "New Global Health Fund – Must be Well Managed if it is to Narrow the Gap Between Rich and Poor Countries." *British Medical Journal* no. 322:1321–1322.

"Risk Groups to be Eyed for AIDS." 1990. *Xinhua General News Service*, January 3.

Rivers, Bernard. 2005. *Consultancy Report: China's CCM – Next Steps (Prepared for and at the request of China's Country Coordinating Mechanism (CCM))*. New York.

Roberts, W. 1998. "Drug Imports on Clinton's African Agenda." *Journal of Commerce*, March 20, 3A.

Rosenberg, Tina. 2008. *Seed Interview: Wan Yanhai*, August 16 2002 [cited March 15, 2008]. Available from http://seedmagazine.com/news/2006/08/seed_interview_wan_yanhai.php.

Rosenthal, Elisabeth. 2000a. "Chinese Media Suddenly Focus on a Growing AIDS Problem." *New York Times*, December 17.

———. 2000b. "In Rural China, a Steep Price of Poverty: Dying of AIDS." *New York Times*, October 28.

———. 2000c. "Scientists Warn of Inaction as AIDS Spreads in China." *New York Times*, August 2.

———. 2002. "China Frees AIDS Activist After Month of Outcry." *New York Times*, September 21.

"Round Table Discussion: Rolling Back Malaria: Action or Rhetoric?" 2000. *Bulletin of the World Health Organization* no. 78 (12):1450–1455.

Rugemalila, J. B., C. L. Wanga, and K. L. Wen. 2006. "Sixth Africa Malaria Day in 2006: How Far Have We Come After the Abuja Declaration?" *Malaria Journal* no. 5 (102)http://www.malariajournal.com/content/pdf/1475-2875-5-102.pdf.

Rutherford, A., A. B. Zwi, N. J. Grove, and A. Butchart. 2007. "Violence: A Priority for Public Health? (Part 2)." *Journal of Epidemiology and Community Health* no. 61 (9):764–770.

Sachs, J. 1997. "The Limits of Convergence: Nature, Nurture and Growth." *Economist (London)* no. 343 (8021): 21–22, 24.

Sachs, J. D. 2001. "A New Global Commitment to Disease Control in Africa." *Nature Medicine* no. 7 (5):521–523.

Sachs, J., and P. Malaney. 2002. "The Economic and Social Burden of Malaria." *Nature* no. 415 (6872):680–685.

Saich, Anthony. 2006. "Social Policy Development in the Era of Economic Reform." In *AIDS and Social Policy in China*, Joan Kaufman, Arthur Kleinman and Anthony Saich. eds., 15–46. Cambridge, MA: Harvard University Asia Center.

Saiget, Robert J. 2002. "Rights Groups Worried at Disappearance of China AIDS Activist Wan Yanhai." *Agence France Presse*, August 30.

Satcher, D. 1999. "The Framework Convention on Tobacco Control – A Report from the 52nd World Health Assembly." *JAMA-Journal of the American Medical Association* no. 282 (5):424.

Sbarbaro, John A. 2001. "Kochi's Tuberculosis Strategy Article is a "Classic" by Any Definition." *Bulletin of the World Health Organization* no. 79 (1):69–70.

Schiller, B. 2000. "AIDS Drug Prices Slashed." *The Toronto Star*, May 12.

Schuman, S. H., S. Olansky, E. Rivers, C. A. Smith, and D. S. Rambo. 1955. "Untreated Syphilis in the Male Negro; Background and Current Status of Patients in the Tuskegee Study." *Journal of Chronic Diseases* no. 2 (5):543–558.

Schwartz, John. 2007. "Tangle of Conflicting Accounts in TB Patient's 12-Day Odyssey." *The New York Times*, June 2.

Schweisberg, David. 1988. "China and AIDS; China Begins to Grapple with AIDS." *United Press International*, March 5.

"Scientist says China has No AIDS 'Sources'." 1988. *BBC Summary of World Broadcasts*, February 3.

Scott, J. C. 1998. *Seeing Like a State: How Certain Schemes to Improve the Human Condition Have Failed*. New Haven: Yale University Press.

Settle, Edmund. 2008. *AIDS in China: An Annotated Chronology 1985–2003* [cited March 15 2008]. Available from http://www.casy.org/chronpage.htm.

"Severe AIDS Effects Seen on Population of Africa." 1996. *The New York Times*, July 3, A5.

Shapin, S., and S. Schaffer. 1985. *Leviathan and the Air-Pump: Hobbes, Boyle and the Experimental Life*. Princeton: Princeton University Press.

Shenon, Philip. 1992. "Edge of the Chasm: AIDS Comes to Asia." *The New York Times*, November 7.

Simons, Marlise. 1996. "H.I.V. Is Still Spreading Rapidly, U.N. Says." *The New York Times*, June 7, A3.

"Sino-American AIDS Symposium Opens in Beijing." 1990. *Xinhua General News Service*, November 8.

Smart, T. 1996. "Nevirapine Surprise." *GMHC Treat Issues* no. 10 (6/7):25.

Smith, I. 1999. "Stop TB: Is Dots the Answer?" *Indian Journal of Tuberculosis* no. 46 (81):81–90.

"South Africa's AIDS Victory." 2001. *The New York Times*, April 20, A18.

"South Africa's Failure on AIDS." 2001. *The New York Times*, June 21, A24.

Specter, Michael. 1998. "Breast-Feeding and H.I.V.: Weighing Health Risks and Treatment Costs." *The New York Times*, August 19, A14.

Stapleton, D. 2004. "Lessons of History? Anti-Malaria Strategies of the International Health Board and the Rockefeller Foundation from the 1920s to the Era of DDT." *Public Health Chronicles* no. 119:206–215.

State Council of China. 1998. The Mid-Long Term Plan of HIV/AIDS Prevention and Control in China (1998–2010). In *State Council Document [1998] 38*. Beijing.

———. 2006. *China's Action Plan for Reducing and Preventing the Spread of HIV/AIDS (2006–2010)*. Beijing.

Sternberg, Steve. 1999. "Victims Lost in Battle over Drug Patents." *USA Today*, May 24, 2D.

Styblo, K., and J. Meijer. 1976. "Impact of Vaccination Programmes in Children and Young Adults on the Tuberculosis Problem." *Advanced Tuberculosis Research* no. 57:17–43.

Sudre, P., G. Tendam, and A. Kochi. 1992. "Tuberculosis – A Global Overview of the Situation Today." *Bulletin of the World Health Organization* no. 70 (2):149–159.

Sui, Cindy. 2001. "Chinese Village Dying of AIDS Neglected and Left to Rot." *Agence France Presse*, March 20.

———. 2002a. "Chinese NGO that Probed Village AIDS Deaths Evicted." *Agence France-Presse*, July 3.

———. 2002b. "Freed China AIDS Campaigner Succeeds in Registering Action Group." *Agence France Presse*, October 18.

Swarns, Rachel L. 1999. "Safety of Common AIDS Drugs Questioned in South Africa." *The New York Times*, November 25, A13.

———. 2000a. "South Africa In a Furor Over Advice About AIDS." *The New York Times*, March 19, A21.

———. 2000b. "South Africa Faults Critics of Its President on AIDS Stance." *The New York Times*, July 11, A3.

———. 2000c. "Mbeki Details Quest to Grasp South Africa's AIDS Disaster." *The New York Times*, May 7, 17.

———. 2000d. "Dissent on AIDS by South Africa's President: Thoughtfulness or Folly?" *The New York Times*, July 8, 5.

———. 2001a. "Study Says AIDS Is Now Chief Cause of Death in South Africa." *The New York Times*, October 17, A5.

———. 2001b. "South Africa May Cite Crisis to Lower Cost of AIDS Drugs." *The New York Times*, March 12, A3.

———. 2001c. "A Move to Force South Africa to Give AIDS Drug for Newborns." *The New York Times*, November 27, A8.

———. 2001d. "Drug Makers Drop South Africa Suit over AIDS Medicine." *The New York Times*, April 20, A1.

———. 2001e. "AIDS-Drug Deal Expected in South Africa Suit." *The New York Times*, April 19, A5.

———. 2001f. "AIDS Drug: Giving the Gift of Life in South Africa." *The New York Times*, February 18, 3.

———. 2001g. "AIDS Drug Battle Deepens in Africa." *The New York Times*, March 8, A1.

———. 2002. "In a Policy Shift, South Africa Will Make AIDS Drugs Available to More Pregnant Women." *The New York Times*, April 20, A8.

Swarns, Rachel L., and Lawrence K. Altman. 2000a. "AIDS Forum in South Africa Opens Knotted in Disputes." *The New York Times*, July 10, A6.

Szlezak, Nicole, and Arnold Howitt. 2004. Generating Multi-Sectoral Collaboration to Combat HIV/AIDS in China: A Local Government Perspective (Poster Presentation). In *XV International AIDS Conference*. Bangkok, Thailand: MEDIMOND S.r.l.

———. 2005a. *Confronting HIV/AIDS in Pingxiang, China (A)*. Kennedy School of Government Case Program (CR-16-06-1785.0): Harvard University.

———. 2005b. *Confronting HIV/AIDS in Pingxiang, China (B)*. Kennedy School of Government Case Program (CR-16-06-1786.0): Harvard University.

The European Mode of Delivery Collaboration. 1999. "Elective Caesarean-Section versus Vaginal Delivery in Prevention of Vertical HIV-1 Transmission:

A Randomised Clinical Trial. The European Mode of Delivery Collaboration." *Lancet* no. 353 (9158):1035–1039.

The Global Fund to Fight Aids Tuberculosis and Malaria (2003). *About the Global Fund – Fighting Aids.* [cited October 5, 2006]. Available from http://www. theglobalfund.org/EN/about/aids/default.asp.

———. 2012. *Framework Document (GFATM/B1/Doc.4)* 2002a [cited January 23, 2012]. Available from www.theglobalfund.org/Documents/core/framework/Core_ GlobalFund_Framework_en/.

———. 2006. *NGOs and Civil Society* [The Global Fund Website] 2002b [cited October 5, 2006]. Available from http://www.theglobalfund.org/en/partners/ngo/.

———. 2006. *Our Development Partners* 2002c [cited October 5, 2006]. Available from http://www.theglobalfund.org/en/partners/international/.

———. 2006. *About the Global Fund – Fighting Aids* [The Global Fund Website] 2003 [cited October 5, 2006]. Available from http://www.theglobalfund.org/EN/ about/aids/default.asp.

———. 2007. *Global Fund Annual Report 2004.* The Global Fund 2004a [cited January 12, 2007]. Available from http://www.theglobalfund.org/en/.

———. 2005. *The Global Fund Website – About the Fund* 2005a [cited August 15, 2005]. Available from http://www.theglobalfund.org/en/about/how/#3.

———. 2005. *Revised Guidelines on the Purpose, Structure and Composition of Country Coordinating Mechanisms and Requirements for Grant Eligibility* 2005b [cited July 2005]. Available from http://www.theglobalfund.org/en/.

———. 2007. *How the Global Fund Works* [Global Fund Website] 2006b [cited January 12, 2007]. Available from http://www.theglobalfund.org/en/about/ how/.

———. 2008. *The Global Fund Website – About AIDS* 2008a [cited February 28, 2008]. Available from http://www.theglobalfund.org/en/about/aids/.

———. 2008. *The Global Fund Website – The Road to the Fund.* The Global Fund to Fight Aids, Tuberculosis and Malaria 2008b [cited May 13, 2008]. Available from http://www.theglobalfund.org/en/about/road/.

———. 2008. *Programs and Portfolio/China.* The Global Fund to Fight Aids, Tuberculosis and Malaria 2008c [cited February 12, 2008]. Available from http://www. theglobalfund.org/Programs/Portfolio.aspx?countryID=CHN&lang=en#.

———. 2012a. "Brochure: Who We Are, What We Do." In *Geneva: The Global Fund to Fight Aids, Tuberculosis and Malaria.* http://www.theglobalfund.org/en/library/ publications/ (accessed January 26).

———. 2012b. *The Technical Review Panel* 2012b [cited January 23, 2012]. Available from http://www.theglobalfund.org/en/trp/.

———. 2012c. TRP Terms of Reference.

Thylefors, B., M. M. Alleman, and N. A. Y. Twum-Danso. 2008. "Operational Lessons from 20 Years of the Mectizan Donation Program for the Control of Onchocerciasis." *Tropical Medicine & International Health* no. 13 (5):689–696.

"Time Running Out for China to Fight AIDS." 1992. *Agence France Presse,* December 1.

"A Total War Against AIDS." 2000. *China Daily*, December 1.

Trigg, P. I., and A. V. Kondrachine. 1998. "Commentary: Malaria Control in the 1990s." *Bulletin of the World Health Organization* no. 76 (1):11–16.

"Triple Therapy in Previously Untreated Patients Reduces Viral Load Below Limit of Detection." 1996. *PR Newswire*, July 9.

"Tuberculosis: A Global Emergency." 1993. *World Health Forum* no. 14 (4):438.

"Tuberculosis: GlaxoSmithKline and TB Alliance Renew Tuberculosis Drug Discovery Program." 2008. *Science Letter*, February 5.

Tucker, J. D., G. E. Henderson, T. F. Wang, Y. Y. Huang, W. Parish, S. M. Pan, X. S. Chen, and M. S. Cohen. 2005. "Surplus Men, Sex Work, and the Spread of HIV in China." *AIDS* no. 19 (6):539–547.

"Two HIV Cases Detected in Yunnan." 1990. *Xinhua General News Service*, November 29.

"U.N. Agency Reports AIDS Virus Spreading Very Quickly in Africa." 1993. *The New York Times*, December 13, B8.

"U.N. Body Appoints New AIDS Director." 1990. *The Toronto Star*, March 21.

"UN to Help China Fight AIDS." 1997. *Xinhua News Agency*, July 9.

United Nations Development Programme. 2012. *UNDP Recognizes Community-Based AIDS Response in China* 2006 [cited January 28, 2012]. Available from http://www.undp.org.cn/modules.php?op=modload&name=News&file=article&catid=14&topic=7&sid=337&mode=thread&order=0&thold=0.

United Nations General Assembly. 2001. *Declaration of Commitment on HIV/AIDS*. New York.

United Nations Joint Programme on AIDS (UNAIDS). 2002. *HIV/AIDS: China's Titanic Peril*. Geneva.

Uplekar, M., and M. C. Raviglione. 2007. "The "Vertical-Horizontal" Debates: Time for the Pendulum to Rest (in Peace)?" *Bulletin of the World Health Organization* no. 85 (5):413–414.

"US Criticised for HIV Aid Effort." 2006. *BBC News*, August 16.

Van Praag, E., K. Kalumba, H. B. Himonga, B. U. Chirwa, and A. Haworth. 1991. "National Aids Control Programs Vertical Vs. Horizontal Approaches the Zambian Case Study." *Istituto Superiore Di Sanita. Vii International Conference on Aids: Science Challenging Aids*; Florence, Italy, June 16–21, 1991. 464p.(Vol. 1); 460p.(Vol. 2). Istituto Superiore Di Sanita: Rome, Italy. Paper:38B.

"VD Cases Multiply in China." 1989. *Xinhua News Agency*, December 2.

Veen, J. 1995. "Drug Resistant Tuberculosis: Back to Sanatoria, Surgery and Cod-Liver Oil?" *European Respiratory Journal* no. 8 (7):1073–1075.

"Venereal Disease in China More than Doubling Every Two Years." 1994. *United Press International*, February 22.

Vergne, L., G. Malonga-Mouellet, I. Mistoul, R. Mavoungou, H. Mansaray, M. Peeters, and E. Delaporte. 2002. "Resistance to Antiretroviral Treatment in Gabon: Need for Implementation of Guidelines on Antiretroviral Therapy Use and HIV-1 Drug Resistance Monitoring in Developing Countries." *Journal of Acquired Immune Deficiency Syndromes* no. 29 (2):165–168.

Verhoef, J. 1994. "The Bcg Controversy." *International Journal of Antimicrobial Agents* no. 4 (4):291–295.

Victora, C. G., K. Hanson, J. Bryce, and J. P. Vaughan. 2004. "Achieving Universal Coverage, with Health Interventions." *Lancet* no. 364 (9444):1541–1548.

Villarino, Margarita E., Lawrence J. Geiter, and Patricia M. Simone. 1992. "The Multidrug-Resistant Tuberculosis Challenge to Public Health Efforts to Control Tuberculosis." *Public Health Reports* no. 1992 (107):616–625.

Von Reyn, Fordham C., and Jonathan M. Mann. 1987. "Global Epidemiology, *In* AIDS – A Global Perspective [Special Issue]." *The Western Journal of Medicine* no. 147 (6):694–701.

Wade, Nicholas. 1988. "Ideas & Trends; Why the Course of AIDS is Defying Africa's Precedent." *The New York Times*, February 21, 6.

Waldholz, M. 2001. "Boehringer, Axios Begin Shipping No-Cost AIDS Drug." *Wall Street Journal*, September 7.

"Wan Yanhai Released after Confessing to Crimes in Leaking State Secrets." 2002. *Xinhua General News Service*, September 20.

Wernsdorfer, W. H. 1991. "The Development and Spread of Drug-Resistant Malaria." *Parasitology Today* no. 7 (11):297–303.

"WHO and China Join Hands in Fight Against AIDS." 1988. *The Xinhua General Overseas News Service*, March 2.

WHO Secretariat. 2008. *The Global Fund's Strategic Approach to Health System Strengthening. Background note 4 for July 30–31 2007 Consultation.* 2007 [cited February 29, 2008]. Available from http://www.who.int/healthsystems/gf22.pdf.

"WHO to Increase Technical Assistance." 1998. *Xinhua News Agency*, August 6.

"WHO Warns China it Faces AIDS Epidemic." 1994. *United Press International*, March 9.

Widdus, R. 2001. "Public-Private Partnerships for Health: Their Main Targets, Their Diversity, and Their Future Directions." *Bulletin of the World Health Organization* no. 79 (8):713–720.

———. 2005. "Public-Private Partnerships: An Overview." *Transactions of the Royal Society of Tropical Medicine and Hygiene* no. 99 (Suppl 1):S1–S8.

Wilhelm, Kathy. 1989. "Law Gives China Broad AIDS-Testing Authority." *The Associated Press*, February 22.

Williams, H. A., D. Durrheim, and R. Shretta. 2004. "The Process of Changing National Malaria Treatment Policy: Lessons from Country-Level Studies." *Health Policy and Planning* no. 19 (6):356–370.

"World AIDS Day." 1988. *Lancet* no. 2 (8617):976.

World Bank. 1993. *World Development Report 1993. Investing in Health.* World Development Indicators. New York.

———. 2008. *The Evolution of the World Bank's Response to HIV/AIDS* 2005 [cited March 22, 2008]. Available from http://www.worldbank.org/oed/aids/docs/report/hiv_chapter2.pdf.

"World Briefing Africa: South Africa: AIDS Drug Sought." 2001. *The New York Times*, August 22, A6.

"World Briefing Africa: South Africa: AIDS Policy Change." 2002. *The New York Times*, April 18, A12.

"World Briefing Africa: South Africa: Order to Distribute AIDS Drug." 2002. *The New York Times*, March 12, A10.

World Health Organization. 1978. *Declaration of Alma-Ata. International Conference on Primary Health Care, Alma-Ata, USSR, 6–12 September 1978* [cited March 1, 2008]. Available from http://www.who.int/hpr/NPH/docs/declaration_almaata.pdf.

———. 1983a. "Acquired Immune Deficiency Syndrome (AIDS) – WHO Meeting." *Weekly Epidemiological Record* no. 58:369–376.

———. 1983b. "Acquired Immune Deficiency Syndrome (AIDS) – Update." *Weekly Epidemiological Record* no. 45:351.

———. 1983c. "Acquired Immune Deficiency Syndrome Emergencies," *Report of a WHO Meeting* (November 22–25). Geneva.

———. 1985. "The Acquired Immunodeficiency Syndrome. Memorandum from a WHO Meeting." *Bulletin of the World Health Organization* no. 63 (4): 667–672.

———. 1989. "Tuberculosis and AIDS. Statement on AIDS and Tuberculosis. Geneva, March 1989. Global Programme on AIDS and Tuberculosis Programme, World Health Organization, in Collaboration with the International Union Against Tuberculosis and Lung Disease." *Bulletin of the International Union Against Tuberculosis and Lung Disease* no. 64 (1):8–11.

———. 1992. "Malaria – Ministerial Conference on Malaria, Amsterdam." *Weekly Epidemiological Record* no. 67:349–356.

———. 1994. *Recommendations from the Meeting on Mother-to-Infant Transmission of HIV by Use of Antiretrovirals*, Geneva, June 23–25, 1994.

———. 1997. *Globalization and Access to Drugs*. Geneva.

———. 1998a. *101st Session of the WHO Executive Board: New Health Policy for the World, New Director-General for WHO (Press Release WHO/16)*. [cited November 18, 2007]. Available from http://www.who.int/inf-pr-1998/en/pr98-16.html.

———. 1998b. *Report of the Ad Hoc Committee on the Tuberculosis Epidemic* (WHO/TB/98.245). London.

———. 2008a. *The Amsterdam Declaration to Stop TB 2000a* [cited March 14, 2008]. Available from http://www.stoptb.org/stop_tb_initiative/assets/documents/decla.pdf.

———. 2000b. *World Health Report 2000: Health Systems: Improving Performance*. Geneva.

———. 2001. *National Health Research Systems. Report of an International Workshop*. Geneva.

———. 2002a. *Global Fund to Fight AIDS, Tuberculosis and Malaria. Note by the Director-General. 55th World Health Assembly (A55/8). Provisional agenda item 13.4*. [cited January 26, 2012]. Available from http://www.who.int/gb/ebwha/pdf_files/WHA55/ea558.pdf.

————. 2002b. *Global Fund to Fight AIDS, Tuberculosis and Malaria. Note by the Director-General. 55th World Health Assembly (A55/8). Provisional Agenda Item 13.4* 2002a [cited January 26, 2012]. Available from http://www.who.int/gb/ebwha/pdf_files/WHA55/ea558.pdf.

————. 2006a. *The STOP TB Strategy (WHO/HTM/STB/2006.37)*. Geneva.

————. 2006b. *Facts on ACTs (Artemisinin-based Combination Therapies)* 2006b [cited March 27, 2008]. Available from http://www.rbm.who.int/cmc_upload/0/000/015/364/RBMInfosheet_9.htm.

————. 2007. *Malaria. Fact Sheet No 94 (May 2007)* 2007a [cited March 22, 2008]. Available from http://www.who.int/mediacentre/factsheets/fs094/en/print.html.

World Health Organization & Joint United Nations Programme on AIDS. 2002. *Accelerating Access Initiative – Widening Access to Care and Support for People Living with HIV/AIDS. Progress Report*. Geneva: World Health Organization. Available from http://www.who.int/hiv/pub/prev_care/en/isbn9241210125.pdf (accessed June).

World Medical Association. 1964. *Declaration of Helsinki: Ethical Principles for Medical Research Involving Human Subjects*. Helsinki.

Wu, Z. Y., S. G. Sullivan, Y. Wang, M. Rotheram-Borus, and R. Detels. 2007. "Evolution of China's Response to HIV/AIDS." *Lancet* no. 369 (9562): 679–690.

Yamey, G., and W. W. Rankin. 2002. "AIDS and Global Justice – Resources from the Global AIDS Fund must Reach the Poorest." *British Medical Journal* no. 324 (7331):181–182.

Yarchoan, R., R. W. Klecker, K. J. Weinhold, P. D. Markham, H. K. Lyerly, D. T Durack, E. Gelmann, S. N. Lehrman, R. M. Blum, D. W. Barry, et al. 1986. "Administration of 3'-azido-3'-deoxythymidine, an Inhibitor of HTLV-III/LAV Replication, to Patients with AIDS or AIDS-Related Complex." *Lancet* March 15; no. 1 (8481): 575–580.

Yardley, Jim. 2007. "Beijing Gives Advocate Praise but No Freedom." *International Herald Tribune*, February 16.

Yusuf, S., S. Ounpuu, and S. Anand. 2002. "The Global Epidemic of Atherosclerotic Cardiovascular Disease." *Medical Principles and Practice* no. 11:3–8.

Zhang, F. J., J. E. Haberer, Y. Wang, Y. Zhao, Y. Ma, D. Zhao, L. Yu, and E. P. Goosby. 2007. "The Chinese Free Antiretroviral Treatment Program: Challenges and Responses." *AIDS* no. 21:S143–S148.

Zhang, Feng. 2002a. "Fight Against AIDS Escalates." *China Daily*, May 27.

————. 2002b. "Ban on Condom Ads Set to Go." *China Daily*, December 2.

Zhang, Fujie, Michael Hsu, Lan Yu, Yi Wen, and Jennifer Pan. 2005. "Initiation of the National Free Antiretorviral Therapy Program in Rural China." In *AIDS and Social Policy in China*, Joan Kaufman, Arthur Kleinman and Anthony Saich. eds. Cambridge, MA: Harvard University/Asia Center.

Zhang, H. X. 2004. "The Gathering Storm: AIDS Policy in China." *Journal of International Development* no. 16:1155–1168.

Zhang, Ke. 2006. *Report on AIDS in Henan after a 5-year Investigation* 2005 [cited March 2006]. Available from www.chain.net.cn.

Zhou, W., Y. Sun, and Z. Wu. 2000. "Acupuncture Ameliorates AIDS Symptoms in 36 Cases." *Journal of Traditional Chinese Medicine* no. 20 (2):119–121.

Zhu, Baoxia. 1997. "China: Steps Taken to Harness Wild AIDS." *China Daily*, November 17.

Index

CPSIA information can be obtained
at www.ICGtesting.com
Printed in the USA
LVHW052327270119
605465LV00008B/407/P

9 781137 020826